Courage to Change

To believe
To hope
To act

To Live!

12 Weeks to Physical and
Spiritual Excellence

Brian Wellbrock

authorHOUSE®

AuthorHouse™
1663 Liberty Drive
Bloomington, IN 47403
www.authorhouse.com
Phone: 1-800-839-8640

First published by AuthorHouse   1/13/2010

ISBN: 978-1-4490-5885-2 (sc)

Library of Congress Control Number: 2009913335

Printed in the United States of America
Bloomington, Indiana

This book is printed on acid-free paper.

Acknowledgments

I would like to thank those individuals who helped bring this amazing project to fruition. First, I thank the Lord for all of my clients over the years who believed in me and my passion for helping them. Those of you I have helped, and will help, inspire me deeply to keep pushing forward in my career and to continue seeking the greatest degree of excellence in my life. I love you all.

Charlie Steinbrueck: Thank you for your support and encouragement as I took a leap of faith into the vast unknown.

Steve and Yvonne Bennet: I love you two and appreciate everything you did for me as I was in the middle of my own *Courage to Change*. Your love and openness as I opened my heart to God's love are a big part of what I now teach and give to others.

Dave and Beth Culler: You opened your home and your lives to me and taught me that one of the most amazing ways to receive God's love is through receiving love and kindness from amazing people like you. Your selflessness and love for each other helped prepare me for this ministry and for my life with Silesia, Shelby, and Matthew. Thank you. I am forever grateful.

Jennifer Burton: Thank you for sharing so much of your energy and time helping research scriptures for the "I Am" section. I AM so proud of you in your own walk with God, your physical health, and restored body image.

Beth Beaulac: (www.beaulacartistry.com) Thank you for your tireless efforts in designing the beautiful title pages and graphics for this entire program. Your gifts in photographic artistry and graphic design are truly amazing. I hope and pray you are blessed beyond imagination for your work with *Courage to Change*.

Scott Philip Stewart, Ph.D.: (www.ScottPhilipStewart.com) *Your* expertise in editing has significantly helped *Courage to Change* become what God intended it to be. Thank you for an amazing job.

My parents Ken and Gladys Wellbrock: Thank you for instilling in me the confidence that I can do anything I set my mind to.

My wife Silesia: You are a part of me and everything I do. I love you.

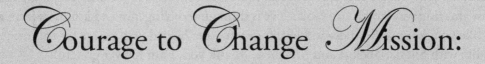

Courage to Change Mission:

1. To lead over 1 million Christians to an exuberant, exciting, amazingly healthy life physically, mentally, and spiritually!
2. To break the yoke of lifestyle induced sickness, disease and infirmity present in the Body of Christ!
3. To lead over 1 million people to the Lord, the foundation of health!

Table of Contents

Foreword . . . . **xi**

Getting Started with Courage to Change 1

- Prologue 3

- Introduction 5

Week 1 7
Setting the foundation by changing the lies and renewing your mind

- Love Notes 9

- Thankfulness 14

- Courage 17

- *The three lacks:*
  Enthusiasm 21
  Motivation 24
  Inspiration 27

- TAP Principle 30

- "I Am" Declaration 38

Week 2 . . . .**89**
How to heal, move forward, and take charge by putting the past behind you

- ASK Principle 91

- Forgiveness 109

- Commitment/Covenant 112

Week 3 . . . . **119**
Setting, reaching, and surpassing your goals and dreams

• Goals 121

Week 4 . . . . **125**
Living as a disciple of Jesus Christ

• Discipline 126

• Obedience 135

• Legalism 145

Week 5 . . . . **153**
Tying in the "I Am" declaration and TAP principle with stress

• Stress 155

• Sleep and Relaxation 161

Week 6 . . . . **171**
The process of change

• Perseverance 172

• The Pain of Love 181

• Fasting 184

Week 7 . . . . **189**
The child in you

• Conquering Fear 191

Week 8 . . . . **201**
A love letter

• Kindness 203

• Conquering Shame 208

Week 9 . . . . **219**
Conquering control and addiction

• Hunger and Thirst 221

• Character 227

Week 10 . . . .**233**
Building relationships by lining up your priorities with God

- Relationships 235
- Compartmentalizing 244
- Law of First Fruits 247

Week 11 . . . .**251**
A call to action

- The Body 253
- Faithfulness 262
- Wholeness 267

Week 12 . . . .**273**
Image of God

- Making Love 275
- Final Encouragement 280

God grant me the serenity
to accept the things I cannot change;

Courage to Change the things I can;
and wisdom to know the difference.

Foreword

From Silesia Wellbrock:

As this book enters its final stage of editing, I realize that all of the thoughts and encouragement that I desire to impart to you must be finalized. The poetic justice of my writing the Foreword is quite comical. You see, I have been an avid reader most of my life (ever since I learned to read), and it has never occurred to me to read the introduction to a book, and while I'm confessing, I usually read the last page first. So, I am asking you to do something that I still struggle with, to please trust the process of this journey. In this book we will laugh, cry, experience anger and weariness, but please know that the heart behind these words is a heart that has such passion for you and your family's health. We want such good things for you and are eternally grateful to be a part of this journey with you.

Yesterday, Brian and I were on exercise bikes at the gym watching HGTV. On the show we were watching as they completely demolished a bathroom. As the cameras spanned the wreckage, I felt myself becoming worried. I looked at Brian and told him how much that panicked me to see the room in such utter disarray. He smiled gently knowing that I am impatient for the finished product. I wish I could bottle that smile for each of you as you embark on the "process" of *Courage to Change*. For you see, that smile says it all to me: "I know this is scary and I know that you are out of your comfort zone, but it really is going to be OK." Sure enough, as it turned out the new bathroom was a sparkling example of what a little effort and a whole lot of demolition can do.

There truly is a story behind the *Courage to Change*. The past few years have been more than filled with all kinds of challenges, including injuries from car accidents, a chronically-ill child, and a couple of hurricanes thrown in for good measure. Making time for our health became a very big challenge for us. I remember telling Brian that if each of you could have 10 minutes in your body feeling optimal health and body weight, that alone would be such a motivation to endure the sometimes painful investments you must make for a healthy body. I wonder how many relationships are wounded simply because a person really just does not feel good physically.

Our society is filled with messages about our weight, what we should eat, and how we should look. The difference in Courage to Change is that Brian allows a sense of freedom and love as you make your own changes toward health. This is not about shame, guilt, or condemnation—but just the opposite! I know how much we love you and want to simplify the steps of living a healthy life.

I love to hear Brian say, "You don't work out to be beautiful, you work out *because* you are beautiful!" Please know—and I mean really *KNOW*—that you are beautiful!!! When you take the time to invest in your health, you are taking the time to love your family and the people around you. I hope that you are so blessed by the stories of our other clients just like you. Pain and trauma may have taken their toll on you, but you can take steps toward healing your body and your soul.

Recently, while watching our son play soccer, my daughter and I were cheering for the team. We didn't know the names of his teammates so his sister asked him to give her a list of the numbers and corresponding names. She and I wanted to root for them by name each time they scored and made a good play. Brian and I want to "root" for you by name, too. I want you to envision the people who love you in the stands cheering you on. Most of all I want you to become a cheerleader for yourself. I am so anxious for you to get to that chapter where...well, I better stop before I give it away. Your race is an amazing one! Next time you get a chance to watch a Nascar race on TV, I want you to notice the pit crew. *Wow*! Everybody on that crew has a crucial job to do for the race to be won! If you were a Nascar driver, who would be on your pit crew? Are you surrounded by healthy people who cheer for you when you make healthier choices? Wherever you are in your race, in this lap, Brian and I are honored to be a member of your crew. We are lining up the tools and ready to jump into action as you rev up the engine with your *Courage to Change.*

Getting Started with Courage to Change

- *Prologue*

- *Introduction*

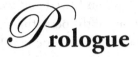
Prologue

Preparing Yourself for Greatness

Be passionate! *How do you express yourself? What are you passionate about?* I'm passionate about life. I love to live! I love to experience life in a way most people only dream about because it reminds me that dreams can become reality. To be great you must believe in your dream and prove the cynics and naysayers wrong, stare down self-doubt and laugh in its face, conquer fear through the power of God, and smile through the better part of every day.

Live in love! Prepare yourself for greatness by going out of your way to do the right thing, or learn something challenging. Express yourself in a new way, or use your imagination at least once a day for something not "work-related." Don't think of Christmas as the only time for love and giving. You can do it all the time, every moment of every day!

Take action! Every step you take should move you closer to the goals you set for yourself. If your steps are not moving you closer, ask yourself and God, *Why am I not moving forward?* And then answer your question with *action*—not words. Talk is cheap; *walk* is not, so act it out! Try this exercise: Live your life as a game of charades. Go a whole day without speaking a word to your loved one and "saying" everything you want to say with actions! Find a way to show "I love you" instead of just saying it. Learn how to make your actions speak louder than words. That is a key to success in *Courage to Change*.

Practice *right*! As you nurture the desire for greatness in every area of your life—personal, professional, physical, sexual, intellectual, and domestic—remember this, it takes practice. A colleague Michael Ditchfield puts it this way, "Practice doesn't make perfect, it makes *permanent!*" Everything in life is an opportunity for learning. So every time you practice something, try to practice smarter than you did before. When I train my clients how to teach their bodies to function properly, it takes a lot of reprogramming to get the old patterns to change. So, we practice. Weeks go by and their bodies slowly develop and change into works of art—not merely because they are practicing, but because they are practicing right! Practicing mastering their body's ability to function, and lose weight, catapults their emotions into fast forward because they feel so good about themselves. They have more energy which allows them the freedom to explore other aspects of greatness.

Have courage! So there's passion, love, action, and practice. But what is the *greatest* requirement of greatness? It is something that you may fear and may take you out of your comfort zone every time. The greatest requirement of reaching personal greatness is having the ***Courage to Change!***

This courage is possible only as you let God transform you from the inside out. Grab hold of his courage and own it for yourself.

Let Jesus take you to the next level! When I lived and worked in Denver, Colorado, I built up quite a booming business. I trained at one of the best athletic facilities in the country—the Cherry Creek Athletic Club. In an average week I would spend 40-55 hours training 75 to 85 people. I would see some of them two or three times a week. I discovered that health facilities and gyms all over the United States had heard of my training and the money I was producing. I was taking people through my original program, teaching, encouraging, and being a mentor to those who wanted help with their health and well-being. On summer weekends, I would take my boat to Lake Granby, high up in the mountains, to enjoy the vastness of the Rocky Mountains.

Though I seemed to have the world in the palm of my hands and was a "great success" in the world's eyes, something was missing. Something inside was telling me that there was another level to my career in training, another level to my calling to help people grow into confident people who were both physically and spiritually mature. My clients were also missing something. Though I had always been a believer in Christ and even talked about God with clients, I felt Him tugging at my heart and telling me that there was something more and that He personally wanted to show me what it was . . . *Him!*

Through His unfailing and unrelenting pursuit of my heart, I found that before my clients could change, *I* **had to change**! I had to learn that even my own health, wealth, and well-being, were not about me, but about Him. So I dropped everything and gave up all I had worked so hard to build and moved to Dallas, Texas. There I spent the next three years in solitude, mostly having the most intimate, mind-blowing, life-altering relationship I had ever been in—my relationship with Jesus Christ. It was a love affair like none other I had experienced. I began writing this book 12 years before it was published. The book wasn't ready until I was ready, and I wasn't ready until I had the *Courage to Change!*

I discovered the principles in this book through my own transformation—a transformation that resulted from surrendering to God's will and calling for my life. This book addresses hundreds of questions from people just like you who have desired physical and spiritual change. I am honored to share this program with you now. I assure you that there is someone who wants to help you become strong and healthy and give you the *Courage to Change.* He is the source of all greatness. His name is **Jesus Christ**.

So may our Lord bless you as you begin this journey. Remember to have fun with life, tap into your potential, be great, and do great things! Don't just take a little nibble out of life! Taste it, savor it, swoosh it around in your mouth, and then, when you have truly felt its texture and tasted all you can taste, gently swallow and demand more! Stuff yourself with *life*, not junk food. Be passionate, strong, and vibrant. Rise to the occasion. Rise to life—and seize the day. Let out a tiger's roar and be heard. Convict yourself with the challenges of personal greatness by having the *Courage to Change* and become strong in the Lord and meet His destiny for you!

Introduction

Let me first commend you on your *Courage to Change!* You are about to learn the value of good health and how to take back control of your life. The way you look at and feel about yourself is about to change *in every way.* As you begin to treat yourself with the respect you deserve, you will experience a boost in your confidence, energy level, and positive attitude. It will open your mind to an entirely new way of thinking. As you learn to love yourself from the inside out, you will take ownership of God's image of you, His **Healthy Image** of you. You will then align your life in such a way as to *be* the amazing man or woman you truly are.

I pray that every word in this book will touch your heart and inspire you to look at your life as one beautiful challenge for personal greatness. I want you to truly learn what it means to be lean and healthy, but, with the right mind, attitude, and actions. As you embark on this wonderful journey of self-discovery and life-change, remember that you can do anything in life you set your mind to so long as you believe in yourself and in others and accept the hand from above to strengthen and lead you. It takes belief, faith, confidence, hard work, and love, love, and more love.

Most of you have started a program and stopped a program, then started a program and stopped a program—rinse and repeat in a vicious cycle. So as you try once again with *Courage to Change,* start off with the belief—the *truth!*—that this time things truly will be different. *You* will be different. You will be changed. This time will be different because you will learn not merely how to eat right and exercise, but how to overcome behavioral and spiritual obstacles that have plagued you for years. Understand that the latest and greatest "magic pill" or "perfect protein meal replacement" is not going to change you. Understand that idolizing male and female fitness models and superstars is not going to change you. Understand that listening to the latest and greatest TV psychologists will not create the changes you desire. The truth is:

Only YOU with the power of GOD can change your life!

Although most people come seeking some kind of change in their physical body, they have had no idea just how *spiritual* the answer is. The fitness and nutrition portion of the *Courage to Change* program is not all that different from many of the other programs on the market. This book isn't *The World According to Brian,* or my wife Silesia, or even certain doctors. It is *The World According to God,* and God is going to make the difference this time because the difference is found in your heart.

Before I go into anything scientific about how to lose weight or exercise, I will dive into your heart, the place where true change begins, the place where God loves you and is waiting to give you the *Courage to Change.* As you probably know from experience, *exercise and eating right* is the easy part. The hard part is *the will to continue,* to keep the commitment you made to yourself and to God to exercise self-control and stay motivated. Together, we will learn how to let God transform your mind and attitude so that you will be able to stay on the path without faltering along the way.

Congratulations! You have already taken the first step!

You have already taken the first step toward changing your life and walking in victory: **You have asked for help!** As we will see in more detail later, reaching out for help out of humility, and a humble heart, is the beginning of life-change because only a humble man, or woman, can really know God, and God is the key to real life-change!

Many of you need extra accountability to take care of yourselves. You need a personal trainer, or coach, standing over you leading the way while you exercise and take care of yourself. For this reason, you may feel weak, insecure, and timid because you cannot "do it on your own." I will let you in on a little secret. By asking for help and knowing yourself enough to understand your weaknesses, you are demonstrating personal leadership and greatness. "**Ask and it will be given to you; seek and you will find; knock and the door will be opened to you. For everyone who asks receives; he who seeks finds; and to him who knocks, the door will be opened**" (Matthew 7:7–8). Your own searching and "asking for help" has brought you to *Courage to Change*.

So get excited! You have just left your old life behind and begun a healthy, courageous journey of self-discovery and life-change with God as your Guide. Be good to yourself always, and have an awesomely healthy day, *every day!* And remember that loving yourself is not conceit. It is a cherished gift from God that you slowly unwrap throughout your life.

So let's get started, shall we?

LAYING the FOUNDATION

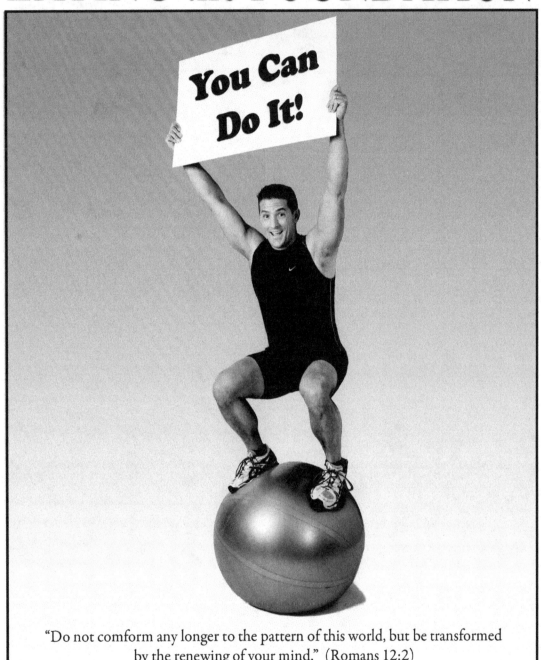

You Can Do It!

"Do not comform any longer to the pattern of this world, but be transformed by the renewing of your mind." (Romans 12:2)

WEEK ONE

$\mathcal{L}$ove Notes

Are you excited? I know I am! I am happy for you and proud to be a part of your journey toward healthy living inside and out. No matter where you are or what your motives are for regaining your health and beauty, the first step is *changing your mindset*. How could you possibly work another program and make healthy changes with the same mindset that got you where you are? Psst… You couldn't. This time will be different. *You* will be different. This program is different. Begin right now looking for God's love notes to you. Let me explain.

One semester in college I was having a rough time. I was depressed and had no idea who I was, or where I was going in life. Despite how I felt, God sent me little love notes to help me through. There were four love notes that really stuck with me.

Love Note 1: "Look up!"

It was a frigid cold January evening, in the second semester of what seemed to be my 25th year of college at Northwest Missouri State University. An ice storm earlier in the day had left everything frozen. I was walking alone back to my dorm room after having dinner at the Union on this cold and lonely night. As I approached the tall prison-like dorm building I looked up and saw one of the most beautiful sights I had ever seen. The two massive trees in front of the dorms were backlit by parking lot lights. I thought my heart would stop. Every limb, every branch, large and small, was perfectly coated with ice and glistened like crystal. It lit up the entire area and sparkled like diamonds. It was like some celestial event had just taken place and I was there to bask in its glow.

I stood gazing up in wonder for quite some time. For most of that semester I had walked with my head down. But God had a love note for me, "Look up!" I believe it was His way of letting me know He was with me and that I should not lose hope.

Love Note 2: "I will never stop pursuing you."

Later that semester, even though much of the snow had melted from the brutal Missouri winter storms, it was still very much wintertime. The gray leafless trees and barren bushes were a good reflection of how I actually felt inside that semester—*dead*. If I was not in class, working out, or eating at the Union, chances were I was in my dorm room sleeping. One day the sun came out, and the temperature warmed up enough for me to open my dorm room windows and let in some cool fresh air. As I lay on my bed staring at the blank wall in front of me, a little sparrow lighted on my window sill to say hello.

It chirped and chirped right next to the window screen. The funny thing was, the bird was looking in at me. It didn't seem at all alarmed and even seemed interested in me. I slowly rose from my bed and went over to the window. Instead of flying away, the little sparrow leaned its head forward with a weird eagerness to communicate. (Did I mention that I was not doing drugs in college… for those of you who might be wondering what I had been smoking!) I put my face right up to the screen so it was not more than three or four inches away from this tiny bird. I watched as its brown eyes blinked and its beak opened and closed as it chirped. I could see its feathers rustle and its tiny little feet steady its footing as the breeze came in.

As I turned my head left, it turned its head left. As I turned my head right, it turned its head right. Its eyes were transfixed on me, and even seemed somewhat enamored. I began to whistle and the little bird stopped to listen. When I stopped, the bird started to chirp. So I listened, then I took my turn and began whistling again. And on it went for 15 minutes. Never once did the bird seem afraid of me and it never moved except to match my moves.

My little sparrow friend finally went about its day, and my spirit was again lifted for a time. I didn't yet know why God would go so far out of His way to get my attention. I would later learn that it was because He loves me. He is the pursuer of my heart and soul, and He will never stop pursuing me.

Love Note 3: "Take heart: Spring is here!"

The third love note came two months later and was, again, unexpected. Though I was doing a little better emotionally, I still wasn't out of the hole I found myself in during that difficult semester. The last snow had melted away, and the warm air seemed to spell the end of winter. The bitter wind that seemed to take a bite out of my skin had changed to a mellow Spring breeze. I had shed my winter coat and could actually walk to class in a long sleeve shirt, or light jacket. My skin, pale and blanched from the frigid winter, welcomed the warm touch of the sun.

It was a magnificent day, yet I looked down, still unable to shake the gloom in my head and heart. I trudged down the sidewalk my feet knew so well as if I was on automatic pilot, not even noticing—much less enjoying—the beautiful day, or my beautiful life.

Once again, though, God was not content to let me hang my head on such a day. He wanted me to look up! He wanted me to be present and actually see and hear the hope and plans He had for me. Halfway to class there was a little hill that led to the Union. It was a real ice hazard after a winter storm, but not this day! A single tree stood right beside the sidewalk. It was the only tree in the entire area. Though still barren from the winter, I could see signs of life in the first Spring buds sprouting green on its branches. As I approached the tree I could hear some commotion. Several other students passing by commented on the disturbance. The closer I came, the louder it got. At the top of this tree was another bird, bigger and louder than the sparrow that had visited me earlier. It was making such a racket that everyone who was walking by noticed. I heard a few comments, "Geez, what's that bird's problem?" and "Shut the #$%$#% up already." As I stopped and listened, my heart began to swell. Students had to walk around me, but I didn't care. The bird obviously had something important to say!

I ignored the other students' comments. I knew exactly what the bird was saying. "IT'S SPRING, IT'S SPRING, IT'S SPRING, EVERYBODY, IT'S SPRING, WAHOOOOOOOOOO!" See, for this bird Spring meant life was being restored from a long, cold winter. It meant the trees were coming back to life, and the once dismal scenery would be lush and teeming with life again. It meant the sun would be warm, food would be plentiful, and the shivering was over. This wasn't just a love note to me and the bird, it was a love note to everyone willing to listen.

For me, it meant the storm was over, my shivering was over! I had survived the cold, dark winter. It reminded me that God brings to life anything that appears dead and even resurrects things that *are* dead. The fresh greenery on the trees represented fresh hope inside of me. I was the tree coming back to life, and the bird was the messenger.

Love Note 4: You are Worth More Than a Test!

A few weeks later, I went to each of my instructors and shared how I had suffered depression throughout the semester. Every single one of them allowed me to postpone my final exam until Fall semester after summer break. After the summer, I came back restored and eager to learn. Not only did I take 21 hours, but I had to finish my classes from the previous semester—all of which were required for me to graduate. But despite all that, for the first time in college I actually enjoyed learning. On my last 12 classes I ended up with nine A's, one B, and one C. And I walked across the stage to receive my diploma with *honor*.

God's Love Notes to You

Friend, know that the storms of life will come and go, and the winters will sometimes seem to wear on forever. Remember that there is a God who loves you and makes all things new. He is always loving you, always pursuing you, and always making Himself known to you. I mentioned how my pale skin from winter welcomed the touch of the sun. What really happened is that the skin of my spirit, pale from the long spiritual winter, welcomed the touch of the SON!

Yes, God's love notes are all around you, wherever you go.

So you might be wondering…. though the fact that God sends us love notes is a wonderful and beautiful lesson, what in the world does this have to do with my health, and why on earth would Brian begin a book on health and beauty with a story like this? I am glad you asked. Listen carefully!

> God came into my realm, on my level, in my space, in the physical world,
> to let me know how important I was to Him.

It isn't just some spiritual experience we have with God as we welcome Him into our hearts. God will make His presence known to you in the physical realm if you will just look. Romans 1:20 tells us: **"For since the creation of the world God's invisible qualities--his eternal power and divine nature have been clearly seen, being understood from what has been made, so that men are without excuse."** God knows we are only human. After all, He made us. He knows we will struggle from time to time, and He will make Himself known to us by what we can *see* if we will only look. He knows it helps us to see His invisible qualities, which the scriptures tell us **"have been clearly seen, being understood from what has been made."** I not only believe in God with the eyes of faith (what I do not see), but by what I *do* see which is *from* Him *to* me in the form of love notes.

See, God loves to show us His beauty, love, and power in the physical world around us. So ask yourself this question, "How much more beautiful to God am I than all of nature, even a perfect diamond or the prettiest bird?" Think about it! He didn't send His son to die for the Rocky Mountains or the Swiss Alps. Jesus did not trade the glory of heaven for the shame of the cross on behalf of the Caribbean or any other exotic and beautiful place on earth. He did it for *whom*? For *YOU!* Nothing is more beautiful to God than YOU! Write this down so you will always remember it that **Taking care of yourself is your way of honoring the beauty that God created in YOU**. You do not train or take care of yourself to make yourself more beautiful or more valuable. You train and take care of yourself because you *are* beautiful and you *are* valuable, even more so than the most beautiful scenery in the universe.

Have you been looking for His love notes to you? They can show up in many forms—a smile from a complete stranger, the early morning dew on a field of prairie grass, or the freckle you love so much on your husband's or wife's arm.

Again, if you will just see God making His presence known by what is seen. Remember Romans 1:20: **"For since the creation of the world, God's invisible qualities--his eternal power and divine nature--have been clearly seen, being understood from what has been made, so that men are without excuse."**

The air you breathe, the beauty you see, and the love you feel inside of you is God's way of letting you experience His love for you *physically*. If you were not physical you could not actually feel anything. Over the next 12 weeks—and for the rest of your life—look for the love notes God sends you every day on your level, in the physical. As you do, it will create in you a deep thankfulness to God for your life, an attitude of gratitude that will permeate all of you, including your health! My prayer is that over the next 12 weeks you will learn that your health, and how you take care of yourself, is a physical love note you send right back to God thanking Him for your gift of life.

For Reflection:

Think back over your life and identify at least three "love notes" God has sent you?

_____

_____

_____

_____

This week, look for—and find—at least two love notes from God to you.

_____

_____

_____

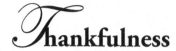hankfulness

"The attitude of gratitude"

Making changes in your behavior over the next 12 weeks will not be easy, but it *will* be easy to let negativity and complaining sabotage your goals!

A smiling heart...

Thankfulness is walking around with a heartfelt smile. Let God teach you to find beauty always in all things and in all people. Look into your heart and thank God for everything—the air you breathe, the sun on your face, your friendships, your job, the car you drive, and the roof over your head. Thank God for His *No's* as well as for His *Yes's.* Thank Him for His holiness, His sovereignty, and for His son Jesus Christ who died and rose again just for you.

Exercise your faith by thanking Him in advance for the things you ask Him for and believing with all hope and certainty that He has given you the answers you seek.

Remember, God's faithfulness is perfect, lacking nothing. Watch how faithful He is to you and how wonderfully He provides the things you need and ask for. Even if His answer is *No,* thank Him knowing that He has your best interest at heart. His sole purpose for you is to prosper you and lead you into a life of true abundance and splendor.

No complaining...

Living with gratitude also means that you do everything without complaining. **"Do everything without complaining, or arguing, so that you may become blameless and pure children of God without fault in a crooked and depraved generation in which you shine like stars in the universe"** (Philippians 2:14–15). How often do you complain about the circumstances in your life? How often do you moan and groan about such menial things as traffic, finances, slow computers, wrinkled shirts, and spilled milk? If you notice yourself having a negative or complaining attitude, just stop right that moment and say, "NO MORE!" Change right then to an attitude of gratitude and "shine like stars in the universe." Immediately thank God for something—for your courage to make changes, for the power in Him you have to change your negative to a positive.

Gratitude brings peace...

The more thankful and grateful you become in all you do, the more peace God will pour into your heart. Ask God to show you how to be thankful in all things, to break the chains of negative, victim-like behavior. As you write in the *Life Application Journal*, share with God—your very best friend—all the things you are thankful for. Go crazy and think of silly things to thank Him for.

Thank Him for the courage He is giving you to take care of yourself and the strength to face positive change with open arms. Thank Him for sharing His wisdom with you throughout the day and providing for your every need. Thank Him for the good, nutritious food you put in your body and the money you had to pay for it. Thank Him for the freedom you have while living in His love and grace. Thank Him for the vast colors in the sky, the wind serenading the trees, and your favorite freckle on your husband's or wife's shoulder. Thank the Lord for from where He has brought you and where He is taking you. He has a perfect plan just for you.

> **"Let the peace of Christ rule in your hearts, since as members of one body you were called to peace. And be thankful."** (Colossians 3:15)

For Reflection:

Right now, look around you and find the beauty in something, then thank God for it!

_____

_____

_____

This week, catch yourself in the act of complaining about something or fault-finding. Stop at once and thank God for some blessing in your life.

_____

_____

_____

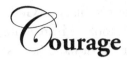ourage

"The Christ-like character that expresses itself in facing danger undaunted; or, in acting despite fear or lack of confidence"

The most difficult part of life-change is embracing and maintaining the right courage and motivation needed to continue taking the right kind of action. So where does your courage come from and how do you get it? Let's find out!

"Be on your guard; stand firm in the Faith; be men of courage; be strong. Do everything in love" *(1 Corinthians 13:14)*. Having the *Courage to Change* is what life is all about. Think of Jesus' courage as He stood in your place and died on a cross for your sins. Like Jesus, we must have the courage to do all things in love.

Courage *Acts!*

Courage of any kind is synonymous with action. Courage that does not act, is no courage at all. And without action, there is no life-change. All of Christ's courage was demonstrated in action, which is the very reason we are saved through His love.

We need to know Christ's love and courage to face our fears. We need to know Christ's courage to be vulnerable with one another. It takes more courage to love than to hate, because to love means to put our hearts on the line just as Jesus did for us. Let us search our hearts for the courage to love one another and to battle complacency and fear. Let us be lifted high by our heavenly father and gain the courage to persevere even while struggling with fear, doubt, and lack of confidence.

Having the *Courage to Change* is just the very first step on the journey to change. You must develop your personal intimate relationship with God and His son Jesus Christ so you can stay inspired and live every moment of your life with enthusiasm.

Over the next 12 weeks in *Courage to Change*, "courage" will actually take on a whole new meaning for you. You will learn that courage is *not* an emotion but a *Christ-like action* that you will take despite fear or lack of confidence. You will learn how to be skeptical when it comes to trusting your own emotions and how to push through them to find a part of you that may have been lost for a while—a part full of strength, perseverance, stamina, and boldness. Acting in courage is required as you have the *Courage to Change*. Old habits, behaviors, and unhealthy lifestyles will be there staring you in the face as you move forward and grow into the healthy person God intended you to be. The good news is that you will face them and conquer them instead of cowering before them, or allowing them to hold you hostage.

Joshua's Courage to Receive God's Blessings

As we consider courage and what it means in this program, let's turn to the book of Joshua. The book of Joshua is about receiving the promises of God. No matter where you are spiritually, *Courage to Change* will equip you with tools to help you navigate through some tough things so that you can eventually step into your "health and fitness promised land"! And just as it was for Joshua and the rest of the Israelites, the land God has prepared for *you* will not just be *given* to you—*you must take it!* Your health is no different! You and God will form a partnership of courage, love, and faithfulness toward one another, and together, you will courageously, aggressively, and proactively take victory in your health, family, relationships, career, and ministry.

If God delivers, why did He repeatedly tell Joshua to be courageous?

So why do you think God repeatedly told Joshua to be strong and courageous? First, because God is always there as your number one fan, the ultimate encourager, coach, mentor, and cheerleader. He will always be inside you speaking life and positive affirmation into you to see that you have everything you need to be successful in your life. Second, God told Joshua over and over to be strong and courageous because Joshua was probably afraid. Let's be honest—Joshua had a pretty big job. He took Moses' place as the military and spiritual leader of millions of people and was called to lead them (who were sometimes more interested in mumbling and complaining than in doing anything constructive) into a foreign land they had to take by force. I have no doubt that Joshua experienced fear, but because of his relationship with God, however, he did not let that fear take root inside of him. Experiencing fear and letting it take root are two very different things.

The act of courage, in spite of fear or lack of confidence, is what breaks and destroys the yoke or root of fear and all unhealthy behavior.

Courage in *Courage to Change* Program Participants

Let me give you a few examples to show what this courage looks like in the lives of some past participants in the *Courage to Change* program. In 2007, I trained a married couple and took them through this entire program. They worked through this book and the *Life Application Journal*, went to my seminars, and made nutritional and exercise modifications—the whole works. A few months into the training program, I noticed a pattern in the wife's behavior during her personal training and exercise sessions that each time I would push her and she would experience muscle fatigue she would get pale, dizzy, and a little fuzzy-headed. Though I considered many possible physical causes for this pattern, I sensed that something else was happening. When I asked her some more personal questions, she confided in me that she had gone through four traumatic, emotionally painful miscarriages. It was difficult for her to even tell me. Tears filled her eyes, and I could see the pain grip her face as she relived the experiences as she told me about them. I pondered how strenuous exercise was related to her past miscarriages. What was the trigger that could bring up these memories on a subconscious level?

During pregnancy, a woman experiences pain, discomfort, nausea, back pain, hormone imbalances, and many other unpleasant symptoms. What makes it all worthwhile is the birth of a beautiful, healthy baby. A woman will willingly endure nine months of physical discomfort to experience the miracle of bringing life into this world. What this woman experienced, however, was very different.

Instead of ending with the joy of welcoming new life into the world, her pregnancies had ended in heartbreak—not once but four times. Thus, she associated physical discomfort with emotional pain and loss. As she realized that the discomfort she experienced during exercise was a memory-trigger for past emotional and physical pain she had a huge breakthrough. As she got to the root of what was happening to her, she began pushing herself more and more. It took tremendous courage for her to continue on through the pain, but she did. It wasn't long before she could go through an entire training session without having those familiar feelings of dread and loss. Those feelings were replaced with hope, and her fear turned to confidence. As she further healed from the loss of her unborn babies, she found courage and learned to embrace the beauty of the process of change called "perseverance." (We will explore perseverance in more detail in Week 6.)

In essence, physical and emotional pains are closely related. As you will find and experience in this book and in the *Life Application Journal*, physical healing leads to emotional healing and breakthrough, and emotional healing leads to physical healing and breakthrough. Each of you has a unique story to tell. Each of you has gone through some "stuff." Over the next 12 weeks you will embrace your courage and learn how to use it in spite of fear, or lack of confidence. As you face physical and emotional insecurities and self-doubt, you will begin to hear God tell you personally: **"Have I not commanded you? Be strong and courageous. Do not be terrified; do not be discouraged, for the LORD your God will be with you wherever you go"** (Joshua 1:9).

As you face fear and patterns of broken commitments, you will begin to hear God speaking to your heart and mind: **"Whoever rebels against your word and does not obey your words, whatever you may command them will be put to death. Only be strong and courageous!"** (Joshua 1:18). Your fear will be put to death. Your poor self-image will be put to death. Your insecurities and sense of worthlessness will be put to death. Your anger and jealousy will be put to death. Your complacency, timidity, passivity, laziness, lack of motivation, and negativity will all be put to death. Anything keeping you from walking in a healthy, action-packed, energetic, exuberant life will be put to death. Even those people in your life who try to bring you down into their own misery and "stinkin' thinkin'", will no longer poison you, and their toxic words will also be put to death.

As you take hold of your courage and put all these things to death, you will hear God speak these words: **"Be strong and courageous, because *you will lead these people* to inherit the land I swore to their forefathers to give them. Be strong and very courageous. Be careful to obey all the law my servant Moses gave you; do not turn from it to the right or to the left, *that you may be successful wherever you go*"** (Joshua 1:6–7).

Who are "these people" God will be speaking to you about? Your family! God will lead you to change your family legacy to one of physical excellence, full of life, health, and energy. You will lead and teach by example. To inherit a legacy of health, means taking action and putting to death old legacies that have not worked. The purpose of this is so "that you may be successful wherever you go." Oh how beautiful is the God we serve!

I am excited for you! Now go and reclaim your health, your life!

> **"Be strong and courageous; do not be terrified; do not be discouraged, for the LORD your God will be with you wherever you go."** (Joshua 1:9)

For Reflection:

Right now, list three things that you feel fearful or insecure about:

_____

_____

_____

What action can you take to exercise courage about each of the things you listed:

_____

_____

_____

This week, catch yourself in the act of feeling anxious, insecure, or fearful. Immediately say out loud: "The Lord God is with me wherever I go." Then take action!

_____

_____

_____

Enthusiasm

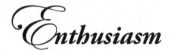

"To be inspired by God"

". . . and your enthusiasm has stirred most of them to action."
(2 Corinthians 9:2)

One day as I was talking with a colleague, he posed the question, "What is it that our clients have desired above all other things as they ask for help?" The answer was threefold. *Enthusiasm* was the first thing. Almost all clients have said at one point or another that they lack enthusiasm regarding their health and well-being. So we decided to look up the word *enthusiasm* in the dictionary. We couldn't believe our eyes. We thought we knew what enthusiasm meant. We, like many of you, thought of it in its familiar sense as "craze, excitement, and a strong liking for something." What we found was that the word *enthusiasm* first appeared in English in 1603 with the meaning "possession by a god." The source of the word is the Greek *enthousiasmos,* which ultimately comes from the adjective *entheos,* "having the God within," which was formed from *en,* "in, within," and *theos,* "God." Over time, the meaning of *enthusiasm* became extended to "rapturous inspiration like that caused by a God" to "an overly confident or delusory belief that one is inspired by God."

How amazing is that!

All that to say that the word *enthusiasm* originally meant "inspired by God." This is important to know because in order for you to change, enthusiasm needs to become an integral part of you. And if you have never been enthusiastic about exercise or eating healthy, then maybe it is the one ingredient that has been missing in your success.

Though I have loved fitness all my life, it was only when I made the connection between health and my faith in God that I understood the true purpose of health in my life. You see, only God's divine inspiration (enthusiasm) can truly change you as you draw Him in. If you are lacking that enthusiasm when it comes to your exercise and eating habits, then you must rely on and ask God to provide it for you. Ask Him to inspire you and He will. If you will involve Him in your daily health and fitness efforts, you will be able to put to rest the complacency that has held you back from using all the amazing gifts God has given you and all the amazing blessings He has waiting for you.

The Faith-Fitness Connection

So many clients over the years have made huge breakthroughs by making the connection between faith, fitness and health, because they learn that their health is a beautiful way of physically expressing their faith.

So start filling your workouts and meals with prayers and praise to God. Live your life with that attitude of childlike exuberance and enthusiasm you once had on the playground with your friends. Choose to stay excited, or "enthused" (inspired by God), and treat each moment as an event to celebrate! It is up to you to choose "in" or choose "out" in life. Don't be indifferent about the health of your body. Indifference is a lack of interest, or concern, an attitude of unimportance, insensibility (lack of feeling), not caring, and listlessness. You don't want that, do you? That is the opposite of enthusiasm and the inspiration of God that will revolutionize your whole life! The choice is yours—enthusiasm or indifference?

"Your faith is made complete by what you do." (James 2:22)

For Reflection:

Think of the last time you were really enthusiastic about anything. What was it? Describe the feeling.

_____

_____

_____

Right now, rate your enthusiasm for making healthy changes on a scale of 1-10:

1 2 3 4 5 6 7 8 9 10

In the space below, write a simple prayer asking God to inspire you to make healthy changes and sign it:

_____

_____

_____

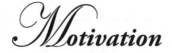

Motivation

"God's Energy"

The second greatest desire people have regarding their health and life in general is *motivation.* Almost every client I have ever worked with has stated in one way or another that he or she lacked motivation. What do you think of when you hear the word *motivation?* Many of you think immediately of something you lack, or want more of, but don't know how to get. What if I told you that there is no one on earth who can motivate you? What if I told you that there is no one thing that can motivate you? You probably think that my next statement is to tell you that only you can motivate yourself. What if I told you that not even *you* can motivate yourself? Even you will let yourself down at times in your life—as most of us have already discovered.

Take heart, for there is one motivator that will never leave you nor forsake you. There is one person who will always have your best interests at heart, one person who will always love you—*no matter what.* That one person is God. Resolve right now to let God be your *only* source of motivation.

God's Energy!

Motivation **in Hebrew means "God's energy."** How awesome is that! Through practice, prayer, and a relentless attitude, you will learn how to turn to God as your source of motivation rather than to magazines that glamorize anorexic young girls, fitness models who haven't eaten a gram of carbohydrates in three months, and people who worship at the Altar of Exercise. The world plays cruel mind games with us, which is why we all—and especially our young women—must go to God for the truth about our value and motivation. Understand this truth: You do not exercise and take care of yourself to make yourself *more beautiful* or *more valuable,* that's backward! The truth is that you take care of yourself because you already *are* beautiful and already *are* valuable. That is motivation!

The root of the word motivation is "motive." God's motive is to work out a perfect plan in your life. You are the one responsible for taking action to accomplish that plan. God plants visions and goals in you, and He will certainly give you the motivation to make them happen. Let *God's* motives become *your* motives. Let *God's* goals become *your* goals. Goals are what keep us moving forward. If we have no goals in life, then it is pretty hard to stay motivated. God certainly will give you a goal to lose weight and be healthy. He already has! Otherwise you would not be reading this. He gives that vision to all of us through His words in the Bible and to each of us personally by His Holy Spirit.

"When you ask, you do not receive, because you ask with wrong motives, that you may spend what you get on your pleasures." (James 4:3)

Asking the "Motive" Question

God knows your heart, your motives. Perhaps in the past you have asked God for more motivation and enthusiasm. Perhaps you have prayed about your exercise and eating habits but feel as though God did not answer you. In times like these, you should ask yourself this question: "What are my true motives for getting back into shape?" Undoubtedly your answer to this question will reveal why you have struggled for so long. Are your motives vain, or are they pure? Are you trying to make your body look a certain way so that you can attract the opposite sex with *the way you look* rather than with *who you really are?* Know this: Feeling attractive, strong, and beautiful is healthy, but it cannot be used as a basis for determining your worthiness in your relationships with other people. Only God determines your value and worthiness!

As God gives you the proper motivation, He will also give you the proper desire. ***Desire* is a Latin word meaning "of the father."** As you go to God for your motivation and your enthusiasm, your excitement will soar to new heights. You will become inspired as God breathes life back into you. His desires become your desires, and His thoughts become your thoughts when you take on the mind of Christ. Jesus Christ had only one thing on His mind—pleasing His father in heaven by knowing His father's thoughts and willingly carrying out His will. Jesus' sole desire was to honor His father, and in doing so He laid down His life for our sins. His desire was "of the father." As you think about the things in your life that you desire, ask yourself how many of them are **"of the world"**, and how many of them are **"of the father."** God knows it is hard for you at times, but as you grow in your love affair with Jesus, you truly take on the desires of God, *including His desire for you to be physically healthy and spiritually mature.*

For Reflection:

What does the following statement mean to you: "You do not exercise and take care of yourself to make yourself *more beautiful* or *more valuable*; that's backward! The truth is that you take care of yourself because you already *are* beautiful and already *are* valuable."

_____

_____

Have you ever tried to motivate yourself? Did it work?

_____

_____

_____

What are your true motives for getting back in shape and working the *Courage to Change?*

_____

_____

_____

_____

Inspiration

"God breathed", or
"Divine guidance, or influence, exerted directly on
the mind and soul of humankind"

The third greatest desire of my clients over the years has been for *inspiration*. They simply have not felt inspired to do anything. Numerous clients have told me, "Brian, I just can't seem to get inspired to haul my sorry behind to the gym or make a commitment to eat good, nutritious food." Could it be that most of us don't have a proper understanding of what inspiration actually is? What inspires you? Can people inspire you? Can things or events inspire you? Yes, all of these things are inspiring, *but the big difference between motivation and inspiration is that motivation can come only from God.* It is something that only He can supply when we look to Him for everything. However, God very much uses other people and events to inspire us, to fill us with hope, and to give us that extra push we need to move forward in our lives. But even though people and events can inspire us, God is right there in the middle of it. Why? What does *inspiration* mean? It means the "act of inspiring", or "breathing." We find the first instance of inspiration in the Bible at the beginning of human history when "God breathed life into Adam."

> **". . . the LORD God formed the man from the dust of the ground and breathed into his nostrils the breath of life, and the man became a living being."** (Genesis 2:7)

Many of you are dying though alive, being choked by the world physically, emotionally, mentally, and spiritually. Let God breathe life back into you. To accomplish anything great, you must first be inspired. Why are you here? Are you here to live with no energy, to suffer from low self-esteem, to have no friends, and to slave away at a job you hate? Absolutely not! You are here to lead, to rule, to take authority in your life, and to live as royalty of the Kingdom of Heaven. Are you getting inspired yet?

We inspire each other as we encourage (empower) one another. We inspire each other as we help and serve one another with love and kindness. We inspire each other as we set out and "do" the things God planted in our hearts. Don't live vicariously through other people's lives. Get inspired yourself and learn to cherish the "doing-ness" of change in your own life. Let people, music, and events inspire you. Listen to something that soothes your soul and inspires you to create something beautiful, then "act" on it and "do" what it has inspired you to do!

Three Key Ingredients

When that inspiration does come along, be careful not to look to the wrong things for motivation. Do you see how it is all intricately connected? To summarize the last few sections, being healthy is a goal, or vision, that God has planted in every one of us. We need **enthusiasm**, the **proper motivation**, and **divine inspiration** to reach that goal. As you begin to journey through this process, you will understand how it all works together as you see evidence of it in your life's transformation, both spiritually and physically.

Finally, as you learn the true definition of these key terms and recall how long you have wanted them, realize that your spirit has been trying to get your attention the whole time. It knows what you need and hungers for the deep things of God. Even as you embark on this wonderful fitness journey, your spirit craves intimacy with God to give you what you need to be successful.

For Reflection:

Do you surround yourself with people who inspire you? If so, who are they? If not, what changes can you make to do so? Where might you find such people?

_____

_____

_____

This week, make it a point to inspire someone in your life by word and/or deed. Who will it be? What will you do?

_____

_____

_____

TAP Principle

"Spiritual alignment: Keeping your thoughts, attitudes, and performance in alignment with God's"

From 1998 to 2001 I lived in Denver, Colorado, one block from the Cherry Creek Trail. The trail ran all through the city and had a wonderful bike path. I would frequently ride my mountain bike on the trail to get my cardio workout in and get away from the hustle and bustle of city things. I often used this ride as a time of reflection. It was a time when just God and I went on a bike ride together. I would often ponder concepts and ideas of how to better my life and the lives of my clients. On one such ride in early summer 2000, my mind was alert and thinking about something one of my clients, a nurse, had said earlier that day during her training session. Between sets we were talking about relationships and what we both wanted in our future mates.

At one point she looked down at the ground, kicked at a piece of equipment, and mumbled, "I just want a man who can make me laugh!" Her voice was low and her facial expression was dark and gloomy. I stared at her for a moment, seeing that something wasn't right. I spoke up, "It probably won't happen with *that* attitude." She looked back at me with that quizzical look I often get from clients when I challenge them. Very gently, I shared with her that her words came out with doubt, pain, insecurity, and negativity. She said she realized that her words expressed her hopelessness because she was doubtful that it would ever actually happen. I shared with her that she would somehow manifest the very thing she didn't want if her thoughts and attitude were full of doubt and hopelessness. She began immediately to change the way she approached that thought. The thought in itself was good. Who doesn't want a mate who has a good sense of humor? But the attitude that followed the thought was one that was already defeated. At some point she had bought into the lie that having a good guy with a sense of humor would never happen to her. For well over a year I helped her change her thoughts and attitudes so they would lead her to act in a way that would bring the future she desired into the present.

On that particular day I did not understand the TAP Principle with the clarity I do today. My experience with that client stayed with me all day, and I thought about it as I rode the Cherry Creek Trail. I thought about how our thoughts and attitude relate to focus and how, sometimes, even though I am looking at one thing, I am focusing on something else. I thought about my attitude and how it affects my performance and actions. All these thoughts were running through my head as I pedaled on around the turns, up and down hills, and around the trees.

About 40 minutes into my ride, as I was on my way back and getting tired, I looked in front of me and saw a difficult turn where the path took me very close to the edge of the drop-off. The path was only a few feet wide and actually ran between a tree and the edge of the drop-off to the creek. I was pedaling pretty hard and took the turn with some speed. As I went around the tree and crept close to the edge, something happened. Now, remember the topics running through my mind were thoughts, attitudes, performance, and spiritual alignment. As I veered around the tree, I looked down over the cliff and instantly became afraid. I leaned hard toward the wide-open field on the other side of the tree and even looked toward the open field, but what do you think happened? You guessed it! Even though I looked at and even leaned toward the open field, I went over the edge of the cliff and plunged eight feet into the shallow creek below.

Ouch!

As I lay there in the creek, I began to take inventory of my body to see if there were any bones protruding through my skin. My bike was on top of my legs and my upper body was on top of my bike. Thank God the creek bottom was sand and not rock. As I realized I was OK and all my bones were in one piece, I began laughing hysterically. Only one thing got broken—my ego. I laughed and laughed out loud as I glanced around to see if anyone had seen me recklessly fly over the edge and free fall into the creek.

I was laughing because I had just proved the entire concept of the TAP Principle: *Our performance always follows our thoughts and attitude*, where our focus is. Even though I was looking at the open field and even leaning toward it, fear was in control of my attitude. My attitude caused me to manifest the very thing I was afraid of, just like my client who had not found a man with a good sense of humor because she didn't believe it would happen. Since that time, I have practiced every day how to keep my thoughts, attitude, and performance in alignment with God. When I let fear penetrate me, I manifested what I was afraid of—falling off a cliff! My thoughts and attitude were not those of power, confidence, and self-assurance, but of fear and doubt. We will discuss fear in greater detail later in this book.

A Young Couple who TAPped into Their Power

So what does this look like for you? How does the TAP Principle relate to you and your goals of taking care of yourself physically, losing weight, exercising, and eating right? In 2002, I worked with a young married couple in Grapevine, Texas. I took them through a four-hour consultation on nutrition, exercise, behavior, the whole nine yards. It was a wonderful session. Both of them let go some amazing things. They went off to work the program into their life and get lean, healthy, and more in control of their health. Wonderful! Except…when I next saw them four to six weeks later, they looked frustrated, beaten up, and at the end of their ropes. They had done everything I asked but hadn't lost any weight. Knowing there had to be a reason, I asked them some probing questions. Turns out, the woman was spending all her time thinking about the foods she used to eat, foods she saw everyone else around her enjoying. At every meal, she would think immediately about something she used to eat. Aha! So she hated what she was doing and resented the changes she was making. Every smell, every sight, and every thought of the foods she used to eat drove her crazy. She approached her exercise the same way—with contempt and a negative attitude. Neither the wife nor the husband had deviated from the program in the least. They even had the "splurge meal" once per week, as I suggest in my program.

What was it? If they had followed my program so closely, why hadn't they lost any weight? Instead of living with the hope, confidence, and victory of Christ, they were unconsciously living in

31

deprivation mode, victims of their own decision to better their health. This couple was a victim of their own program. They were living in the past, allowing their old habits, cravings, and urges to take control of them rather than taking control over their lives with a strong, confident attitude. They were letting food control them rather than control food through their thoughts and attitudes. They both said that they felt whipped, and why wouldn't they? They had given all their control away.

During that second time I saw them, I was gentle, yet very stern. I shared with them how the enemy was influencing their thoughts and attitude with negativity, doubt, frustration, and failure. In essence they were giving the enemy permission to torment them with counterproductive thoughts and attitudes that would accomplish the enemy's goal of keeping them far from reaching *their* goal. I shared with them that it was up to them to take captive their thoughts and to make them obedient to Christ. No one would do it for them. I asked them, "Have you ever thought of how bizarre it is that you give 'food' power over you? Or anything else for that matter. How can food have power over you when it is *you* who consume *it*? Wasn't this world created for you to lead and to rule with love and peace? Why would you relinquish your control like this and let the world dictate your joy and happiness? It is you who are in control over food, your behavior, thoughts, attitudes, actions, and everything else in your life." I shared a few scripture verses with them and encouraged them to claim God's truth in their own lives:

"Forget the former things; do not dwell on the past." (Isaiah 43:18)

"Brothers, I do not consider myself yet to have taken hold of it. But one thing I do: Forgetting what is behind and straining toward what is ahead, I press on toward the goal to win the prize for which God has called me heavenward in Christ Jesus." (Philippians 3:13–14)

As I shared these scriptures and spoke this truth about where their thoughts were coming from, the wife actually got angry, not at me, or herself, but at the enemy. Once she realized she was being controlled, her facial expression changed, her countenance changed, and her entire demeanor changed. She looked at me with bold, heated eyes and said to me, "You mean to tell me that I have allowed myself to be influenced this whole time, and that is why I have been so miserable?" She was flat ticked off. I hadn't even told her that was what it was. I simply asked her if these feelings of hopelessness and despair were feelings God would give her. She knew the answer was *No* and realized instantly where they were coming from. The husband just stood there shaking his head as he realized what had been happening to them.

So what happened next? They were inspired as God breathed life back into them. I think what God really breathed into them was fire because they left with a renewed strength and the attitude of a warrior ready for battle. They realized they had to start relying on God for their strength and *Courage to Change*. By the time I next saw them seven weeks later they had both lost 20 pounds and were glowing with good health. They were walking tall and proud. They were in charge. They were confident in the power of God working in them and knew where their strength came from. They had experienced firsthand how powerful their mind and attitude were when they were led by hope and the authority of Jesus Christ. Each time I saw them after that, they both shined like lights because they had learned how to take control of and use their thoughts and attitudes as weapons to regain their authority.

The amazing thing about this story is that their performance (action) was right on target. They were doing exactly what they were supposed to be doing the whole time. But though their actions changed, the results followed their thoughts and attitude. All three—thoughts, attitude, and performance—must be in alignment with God to get results and maintain them. They put the past behind them and even ate junk food once in a while. But they became responsible and controlled when and how much. They basically told the enemy where to go and began living their lives with the hope and peace of Christ! Shortly after meeting this couple, I began developing the "I Am" section of this book.

As with me on the Cherry Creek Trail, you will have to navigate your way beside many cliffs throughout your life. You will plunge over some of them and overcome others. God will protect you regardless. When you put these principles into practice, they can and will set you free. Take captive your thoughts, live with a positive Christ-like attitude, and do (perform) as Christ would.

How to Understand and Apply the TAP Principle

The only way you can become physically and spiritually mature is to have daily fellowship with God. This maturity is the foundation that allows you to balance your life mentally, emotionally, and physically. Each morning you must TAP into alignment, which means that you align your *t*houghts, *a*ttitudes, and *p*erformances with the word of God.

Prepare yourself each morning for a day of blessed events and love. God not only loves you, but He likes you, and wants to be with you even more than you want to be with Him. When you invite God to spend each moment with you He will bless your every move. Christ is the "Great I Am," He is not the "I Was", or the "I Will Be." First thing each morning you must get right with Him, then live moment-by-moment with courage and enthusiasm.

The basis of this whole program is that you "DO" three things daily:

1. Be responsible and, first thing every morning, take ownership of your thoughts, attitude, and performances (TAP).
2. Live in the moment (NOW)
3. Reflect (review your performance at the end of each day)

1. Morning TAP In!

"Very early in the morning, while it was still dark, Jesus got up, left, and went off to a solitary place, where he prayed" (Mark 1:35). The first half hour of the day sets your day in forward motion. It is the rudder of your day. After you read the Bible, you should fill out the "Act as if . . ." page in your *Courage to Change Life Application Journal.*

Avoid reading the newspaper or watching television. The first 30–60 minutes should be between you and God only. Television and newspapers program your mind and emotions with **"Sin**sationalism," external stimulation, power, money, greed, violence, and sexual immorality.

What you want to program your mind and emotions with is "**Son**sationalism," inner peace, hope, love, and gentleness through Jesus Christ. You must get right with God before you do anything. Watch and be amazed.

First, read the Bible

The Bible is alive! Every word lives inside of us. It is the most inspirational, motivational, and educational book ever written. The Bible educates us on pain, suffering, and hardships that come in this life and how to persevere and overcome all difficulties. The Bible is the most positive and encouraging instrument for life-change ever written. The Bible not only reveals how we get saved but serves as the blueprint for how we can live our lives more abundantly.

Second, TAP in and pray: Journaling

As it is written, so shall it be done! The write-it-down process is the precursor to all other actions because our thoughts and prayers are brought to physical reality as we write them down. How can we do what we need to do for God if we keep everything in our heads? We can't! So let it out. Write it down and free your mind of all things except positive thoughts inspired by the word of God.

After your morning TAP, you must stay TAPped in to each moment for the rest of the day. How? By controlling your thoughts, maintaining your childlike attitude, and performing (all that you do) with enthusiasm. On those days when you have difficulty fitting everything in, **be sure at least to journal** and then find time throughout the day to read your Bible.

Thoughts

"And we take captive every thought to make it obedient to Christ" (2 Corinthians 10:5). Everything any man or woman ever accomplished began as a single thought. That's why you have to align your thoughts with the truth. If you are not in the word of God, your thoughts will keep you from living with self-control and enthusiasm. When you write down positive thoughts, you become more conscious of them. Journaling positive thoughts in the daily "Act As IF" portion of the *Life Application Journal* is an extremely effective way to **be transformed by the renewing of your mind** (Romans 12:2). Dr. Norman Vincent Peale wrote, "Positive thought is a synonym for Faith." If and when you notice a negative thought entering your mind, make a shift and change it to something positive. Don't indulge a negative thought for one moment! In the days, weeks, months, and years to come, you will change your thoughts to powerful, confidence-building, positive affirmations that keep you inspired and encouraged all day long. Writing positive thoughts and affirmations first thing in the morning programs your mind for a day of victory.

Attitude

"Your attitude should be the same as that of Christ Jesus" (Philippians 2:5). Attitude is everything...*almost.* If what you think about is not followed by a positive attitude, you will never achieve the abundance God has in store for you. If your attitude, or emotional state, regarding something you do not have or want is negative, it is an insult to God. God created you and your healthy desires, and He will give you those desires so long as you ask in faith. **"May he give you the desire of your heart and make all your plans succeed"** (Psalms 20:4).

Negativity and doubt express a lack of faith. The way to overcome a negative circumstance is with positive thoughts, or faith. Every one of us experiences negative circumstances at some point in our lives. They are a part of life. What enables us to overcome them is our thoughts and attitudes. Are you a victim in life or a **"response-able"** Christ follower? The choice is yours. Your attitude will dictate how you respond to any given situation. If your attitude is negative, your response will always be negative and your desires will remain in the "unattainable" future. But when you think positive thoughts (faith), they will lead to positive attitudes and emotions, and you immediately bring the future of what you want into the present. That is when you begin to truly TAP into God's abundance.

Performances

"Dear children, let us not love with words or tongue but with actions and in truth" (1 John 3:18). Being in alignment with God means letting your positive thoughts and attitudes lead you to perform actions and deeds that honor Him. Think of the action that you do, or do not, take as obedience or disobedience. Once you bring the future of what you want into the present by creating positive thoughts and attitudes, the actions that follow are what produce abundance. Remember, **"Your faith is made complete by what you do."** The only way to pick an apple from a tree is by physically taking action and grabbing one. The fruit of your life is no different. The only way you can harvest what God wants for you is to *ask* him for the correct positive thoughts and attitude and then take the action necessary to fill up your basket. No one will do it for you. Not even God will do it for you. You are **"response-able"** for all of your actions in your life.

2. Live in the Moment (NOW)

Where have you been living—in the past or the future? It is pretty hard for us to fathom eternity because we think of time as a definite (or finite measurement) on earth. We think of time as minutes, hours, or days. The power of now is puzzling, yet freeing, because *now* is where you realize that God and eternity are. Now is where God is waiting for you to love Him and be loved by Him. So many of you are living in the past or the future. If you live with guilt, shame, resentment, blame, unforgiveness, or condemnation, you are living in the past. If you live with any kind of fear at all, you are living in the future. In the Bible, Paul teaches us the proper perspective on our past, **"Forgetting what is behind and straining toward what is ahead, I press on toward the goal to win the prize for which God has called me heavenward in Christ Jesus"** (Philippians 3:13–14). We are also taught about the future when we read, **"'For I know the plans I have for you,' declares the LORD, 'plans to prosper you and not to harm you, plans to give you hope and a future'"** (Jeremiah 29:11). This knowledge about forgetting our past and being assured of the promise we have of a prosperous and hopeful future makes it much easier to live in the now!

So are you going to think about all the times in the past when you started a diet and exercise program and failed? No! Are you going to think about the gloom of another failure with this program? No! With the grace of God you are going to start this program right now because "you are the program"!

3. Evening Reflection

During your evening reflection time, you will learn whether you are, or are not, doing the deeds and performing according to His will.

"Do not let the sun go down while you are still angry, and do not give the devil a foothold" (Ephesians 4:26–27). The last 15 minutes of the day is what prepares you for a restful sleep and sets the tone for the next day. You want your life to be in forward motion. Your *Evening Reflection* in the *Captain's Log* and journaling in the *Life Application Journal* clear the air of your day, teach you where your successes and struggles were, and provide a clean slate for the next morning's TAP in session with God. Every day is a new day. When your head hits the pillow, you must be right with God so that you will not carry all the baggage into the next day, and thus, never move your life in forward motion. Never go to bed with any kind of negative emotion, or stress, from your day. If you don't reflect on your day and get right with God, you will end up using the next morning to clean up the previous day's messes, which sets you back!

Reflect on all areas of your life to be right with God because He is the foundation of everything you do. Your life has many components. Through recording your reflections in your journals in the following days, weeks, and months, you will expose where you are, and are not, balanced in each component of your health.

For Reflection:

Commit this principle to memory: **TAP Principle:** *Our performance always follows our thoughts and attitude*

_____

_____

_____

This week (and every week), catch yourself in the act of entertaining a negative thought, or bad attitude, and stop the devil in his tracks. Immediately, affirm God's truth about the situation or event.

_____

_____

_____

"*I*AM *D*eclaration"

"Owning or appropriating the truth about what God says about you"
"The single greatest tool on earth for life change."

For years in church I heard that I was to *take my thoughts captive and make them obedient to Christ and have the attitude of Christ.* I always got excited and inspired as I heard gifted Holy Spirit–filled preachers talk about the renewing of the mind through God's word. But I always wondered how am I supposed to do this? What does it look like to "take captive my thoughts and make them obedient to Christ"? I got all excited about this principle, but I didn't know or understand how to apply it in my own life. How and where did it show up in my life, and what role did I play in the renewal of my mind as I dived into God's word? I kept asking these questions because I didn't want merely to be inspired by great messages. I wanted to apply the principles and work them! I wanted change!

As I asked questions and sought answers, God began teaching me about ownership, authority, and just how powerful His love really is. You are about to learn how to take these concepts to a new level by taking ownership of the truth and power of God. **Once you realize who you are, who you serve, and the rights you have, you, like me, will begin to live your life with confidence, boldness, and self-control, and will take back what is rightly yours and live daily in the authority of God.**

Jesus restored your authority and inheritance here on earth when He fulfilled the law, died on the cross, rose again, and poured out His Spirit. The problem many of us face is that we do not have the slightest idea how to recapture this authority for ourselves. It is not enough merely to know God's word. We must appropriate, or take ownership of, God's word and truth for ourselves in our own lives. **"For in Christ all the fullness of the Deity lives in bodily form, and you (YOU) have been given fullness in Christ, who is the head over every power and authority"** (Colossians 2:9–10). This must become a part of you, written in your essence. It must drip from your tongue and permeate everything you do. Your spirit knows and craves this truth and is there to help you and guide you.

God's Truth vs. the Enemy's Lies

You have been given "fullness in Christ" and must learn to identify and contradict the negative beliefs, or lies (in the form of thoughts), that violate your spirit and the word of God. The "truth" is the antidote to the lies the enemy tells you about yourself. How can you possibly take care of yourself and be healthy if you are insecure and timid and think that what you see in the mirror is horrific, ugly, or disgusting? Do not ever take ownership of negative thoughts and limiting beliefs like these because they do not come from you…and they certainly do not come from God. You must take responsibility for how you respond to these thoughts and beliefs, but realize that they are not your own. You would never purposely sabotage yourself. The enemy constantly plants seeds of doubt, pain, worry, stress, fear, and anger in your mind. This is how he tempts you and deceives you. Sometimes those words come from people who are supposed to be close to you and love you. I think the enemy does his best work this way. Do *not* let the words or thoughts take root. Whenever you have a negative thought, or a limiting belief stirs within you, immediately admonish, or reverse, it in the name of Jesus Christ. Remind yourself of the truth, which is the opposite of what the enemy is telling you. The weapon you need to fight with to defeat the enemy and take back your authority is this: a constant reminder of who Christ says you are!

"Resist the devil and he will flee from you." (James 4:7)

The "I Am" is the single greatest tool for life change. Your actions usually follow your belief system. "I Am" involves ownership of a thought, or attitude, either positive or negative. It is your belief system. Even if you change your actions, you can still be controlled through your thoughts and attitude. Even though you have changed your behavior (actions), fear and resentment can still haunt you. How many times have you begun an exercise and nutrition program only to get hit with a barrage of thoughts of insecurity, inability, weakness, doubt, hopelessness, and so you quit? The "I Am" gives you power over all thoughts and attitude in *every* area of your life.

When Jacob left Beersheba and set out for Haran, he stopped to sleep for a while and had a dream. **"He had a dream in which he saw a stairway resting on the earth, with its top reaching to heaven, and the angels of God were ascending and descending on it. There above it stood the LORD, and He said: 'I AM the LORD, the God of your father Abraham and the God of Isaac'"** (Genesis 28:12). God first had to know who He was to approach Jacob with that introduction. Then God let Jacob know who was talking to him. Once He told Jacob who He was and got his attention, He told Jacob, **"I will give you and your descendants the land on which you are lying. Your descendants will be like the dust of the earth, and you will spread out to the west and to the east, to the north and to the south. All peoples on earth will be blessed through you and your offspring"** (Genesis 28:13–14). God told Jacob who He was because He knew that thoughts and dreams from the enemy, full of lies and trickery, influenced Jacob all the time, just as they do us. When you are given a thought that is not in alignment with God, you must first do as God did here with Jacob and tell the thought who you are. God told Jacob **"I AM the Lord."** Do you know who you are? Once you have stated who you are with confidence and dignity, then give the command, or instructions, just as God did with Jacob. The reason Jacob listened and did what God said was that it was *God* who was talking to him. You have this same authority over your thoughts when they are in violation of the truth. When you state who you are and who you serve (Jesus Christ) you will get the enemy's attention immediately. And He must listen and do as you say.

Notice that before God says "I WILL" give you and your descendants the land, he starts with "I AM" the Lord! "I WILL" states a promise in the future. But the **"I AM"** is the action fulfilling what the **"I WILL"** promised. Since God is the Great **"I AM"** and is perfect, the **"I AM"** *always* follows the **"I WILL"** (or promise). So don't get caught up in the **"I WILL"** because it only means that you haven't done anything yet! It is simply a promise you need to fulfill with the

"I AM." Which of the following two statements shows what you are currently doing—"I WILL" exercise and eat right, or, "I AM" exercising and eating right? Where have you been spending your time—in the I WILL or in the I AM? The "I Will" is discussed in more detail in week 3.

Many Christians consider their negative thoughts as simply a belief system and are afraid to explore where they came from. If you don't understand the origin of these beliefs, or lies, you will never truly have authority in your life. After all, why did Jesus die for you in the first place? He died to secure your salvation *and* to *restore your authority over the enemy here on earth*. Yes, there is an enemy, but you have been given authority over him.

It is up to you to exercise this authority with the "I Am."

Women, don't for a minute let the word *authority* intimidate you or turn you off. You have the very same authority over the enemy as any man, and it is high time you start using it. How awesome is that!

As a recap, you must do four things to change a lie or belief to the truth:

1. **Address** the thought and the one who is telling it to you (the enemy) with the **"I Am"** by confidently and knowingly stating *who you are* and *who you serve*.
2. **Command** the thought and the enemy to leave in Jesus' name.
3. **Change the lie** and contradict it with the truth in God's word, beginning with the "I Am."
4. **Validate** the change with God's word.

Many of my clients have overcome the following negative thought, or lie, so I will use it to demonstrate how to take these four steps.

Believed lie: "I am unworthy"

1. **Address:** "I AM" a son or daughter, a King or Queen, and heir of the most high God and "I AM" a servant of the Lord Jesus Christ. **Say it with power!**
2. **Command:** "I AM" commanding you, the enemy and thought of unworthiness, to leave in Jesus' name. You have no authority here or anywhere else in my life. **You are pond scum beneath my toes! Say it with more attitude this time!**
3. **Change the lie:** "I AM WORTHY!" Mean it!
4. **Validate:** "I AM" so worthy that I am" "**given authority to trample on snakes and scorpions and to overcome all your power Satan; nothing will harm ME**" (Luke 10:19). "I AM" so worthy that "**For God so loved ME that he gave His one and only Son, that when I believe in Him I shall not perish but have eternal life**" (John 3:16). "I AM" so worthy that "**He will never leave me nor forsake me**" (Deuteronomy 31:6).

How can you actively take care of yourself and be healthy with joy and peace—or do anything, for that matter—when you believe the lie that you are unworthy? In number 4, you aren't changing scripture. You are simply applying the truth to your life by taking ownership of the truth yourself!

> **"Jesus answered, 'I AM the way and the truth and the life.'"** (John 14:6)

> **"'I AM the Alpha and the Omega,' says the Lord God, 'who is, and who was, and who is to come, the Almighty.'"** (Revelation 1:8)

Jesus knows who He was, who He is, and is to come! As His follower, you can do this with the certainty that God's truth is not something you simply know and can recite, but rather something you own for yourself and claim with confidence, fervor, passion, and total conviction!

> **"We demolish arguments and every pretension that sets itself up against the knowledge of God, and we take captive every thought to make it obedient to Christ."** (2 Corinthians 10:5)

Following is a list of beliefs, or lies, that we all have battled with from time to time. I have helped clients identify and overcome every one of these lies. This entire list has come from clients I have worked with—people just like you. Every one of these lies is a direct violation of your spirit and the word of God. And you wonder why you have had trouble being motivated to do anything! **Remember that your actions must always follow your changed belief!** If they don't, then you really didn't change your belief to the truth because truth is always accompanied by action. Take hold of who you are, of who God says you are, and take back your authority and own the truth of God for yourself. Your life depends on it!

Lie	Truth	Validated by God's Word
I am fat I am disgusting I am ugly I am repulsive	I am radiant I am beautiful I am handsome I am lovely I am elegant I am accepting of my body now	• "For you created my inmost being; you knit me together in my mother's womb. I praise you because I am fearfully and wonderfully made; your works are wonderful, I know that full well." (NIV Psalm 139:13-14) • "How beautiful you are, my darling! Oh, how beautiful! Your eyes are doves. How handsome you are, my lover! Oh, how charming! And our bed is verdant." (NIV Song of Solomon 1:15-16) • "I am a daughter of the king, I am among His honored women. The king is enthralled by my beauty; I am honoring Him because He is my lord. I am glorious within my chamber, I am led with joy and gladness as I enter the palace of the king." (NIV Psalm 45:9,11,13,15) • "I delight greatly in the LORD; my soul rejoices in my God. For he has clothed me with garments of salvation and arrayed me in a robe of righteousness, as a bridegroom adorns his head like a priest, and as a bride adorns herself with her jewels." (NIV Isaiah 61:10)
I am inferior I am not good enough	I am royalty I am an heir I am a friend of God I am equal!	• "I am a son or daughter, God sent the Spirit of his Son into my heart, the Spirit who calls out, Abba, Father. So I AM no longer a slave, but a son or daughter; and since I AM a son or daughter, God has made me also an heir." (NIV Galatians 6,7) • ". . . so that there should be no division in the body, but that its parts should have equal concern for each other. If one part suffers, every part suffers with it; if one part is honored, every part rejoices with it. Now you are the body

Lie	Truth	Validated by God's Word
	I am good enough	of Christ, and I AM a part of it." (NIV 1 Corinthians 12:25-27) • "For God so loved me that he gave his one and only Son, that when I believe in him I shall not perish but have eternal life." (NIV John 3:16)
I am poor **I am broke**	**I am wealthy** **I am prosperous**	• "While in my humble circumstances I am taking pride in my high position." (NIV James 1:9) • "I am submitting to God and I am at peace with him; in this way prosperity will come to me." (NIV Job 22:21)
I am average **I am below average**	**I am anointed** **I am gifted**	• "As for me, the anointing I received from him remains in me, and I do not need anyone to teach me. But as his anointing teaches me about all things and as that anointing is real, not counterfeit—just as it has taught me, I remain in him." (NIV 1 John 2:27) • "Now it is God who makes me stand firm in Christ. He anointed me, set his seal of ownership on me, and put his Spirit in my heart as a deposit, guaranteeing what is to come." (NIV 2 Corinthians 1:21-22) • "Every good and perfect gift I have is from above, coming down from the Father of the heavenly lights, who does not change like shifting shadows." (NIV James 1:17)

Lie	Truth	Validated by God's Word
I am afraid	I am courageous I am bold I am strong I am faith filled	• "I am strong and courageous, not terrified, or discouraged, for the LORD my God is with me wherever I go." (NIV Joshua 1:9) • "The LORD is my light and my salvation—whom shall I fear? The LORD is the stronghold of my life—of whom shall I be afraid?" (NIV Psalm 27:1)
I am angry	I am kind I am gentle I am peaceful	• "In my anger I do not sin: I do not let the sun go down while I am still angry, and I do not give the devil a foothold." (NIV Ephesians 4:26-27) • "I am quick to listen, slow to speak and slow to become angry, for my anger does not bring about the righteous life that God desires." (NIV James 1:19-20) • "But the fruit of the Spirit is love, joy, peace, patience, kindness, goodness, faithfulness, gentleness and self-control. Against such things there is no law. Those who belong to Christ Jesus have crucified the sinful nature with its passions and desires. Since I live by the Spirit, let me keep in step with the Spirit." (NIV Galatians 5:22-25)

Lie	Truth	Validated by God's Word
I am unworthy	**I am worthy**	• "I am (was) created to rule over the fish of the sea and the birds of the air, over the livestock, over all the earth, and over all the creatures that move along the ground." (NIV Genesis 1:26) • "For God so loved ME that he gave his one and only Son, that when I believe in him I shall not perish but have eternal life." (NIV John 3:16) • I AM worthy enough that, "He will never leave me nor forsake me." (NIV Deuteronomy 31:6)
I am a loser **I am worthless**	**I am a winner** **I am glorified** **I am priceless**	• "And I know that God works for my good because I love him and I am called by him according to his purpose. God foreknew me and predestined me to be conformed to the likeness of his son, that he might be the firstborn among many brothers. I am predestined by him, and also called by him; I am called by him and also justified by him; I am justified by him and also glorified by him." (NIV Romans 8:28-30) • "What, then, shall we say in response to this? If God is for me, who can be against me?" (NIV Romans 8:31) • "My Life is more than food, and my body more than clothes. Consider the ravens: They do not sow or reap, they have no storeroom or barn, yet God feeds them. And how much more valuable Am I than birds!"

Lie	Truth	Validated by God's Word
I am lazy I am complacent	I am energetic I am a doer	• "I pray that out of his glorious riches he may strengthen me with power through his Spirit in my inner being, so that Christ may dwell in my heart through faith. And I pray that I, being rooted and established in love, may have power, together with all the saints, to grasp how wide and long and high and deep is the love of Christ, and to know this love that surpasses knowledge—that I may be filled to the measure of all the fullness of God." (NIV Ephesians 3:16-19) • "I am pressing on toward the goal to win the prize for which God has called me heavenward in Christ Jesus." (NIV Philippians 3:4) • "For God did not give me a spirit of timidity, but a spirit of power, of love and of self-discipline." (2 Timothy 1:7)
I am envious	I am a peacemaker I am secure in my good standing I am content in the Lord	• "For where you have envy and selfish ambition, there you find disorder and every evil practice. But the wisdom that comes from heaven is first of all pure; then peace-loving, considerate, submissive, full of mercy and good fruit, impartial and sincere. Peacemakers who sow in peace raise a harvest of righteousness." (NIV James 3:16-18) • "My fear of the LORD leads to life: I am resting content, untouched by trouble." (NIV Proverbs 19:23)

Lie	Truth	Validated by God's Word
I am un-motivated	I am motivated I am willing	• "Then the sovereignty, power and greatness of the kingdoms under the whole heaven will be handed over to me, a son or daughter of the Most High. His kingdom will be an everlasting kingdom, and I will worship and obey him." (NIV Daniel 7:27) • "Wash away all my iniquity and cleanse me from my sin." (NIV Psalm 51:2) • "Therefore, I endure everything for the sake of the elect, that I too may obtain the salvation that is in Christ Jesus, with eternal glory. Here is a trustworthy saying: If I died with him, I will also live with him." (NIV 2 Timothy 2:10-11)
I am uninspired	I am inspired	• "All scripture is given by inspiration of God, and is profitable for doctrine, for reproof, for correction, for instruction in righteousness. That I, a man or woman of God, may be perfect, thoroughly furnished unto all good works." (KJV 2 Timothy 3:16-17)
I am dumb	I am wise I am brilliant I am smart	• "If I lack wisdom, I should ask God, who gives generously to all without finding fault, and it will be given to me." (NIV James 1:5) • "God's purpose is that I may be encouraged in heart and united in love, so that I may have the full riches of complete understanding, in order that I may know the mystery of God, namely, Christ, in whom are hidden all the treasures of wisdom and knowledge. God tells me this so that no one may deceive me by fine-sounding arguments." (NIV Colossians 2:2-4)

Lie	Truth	Validated by God's Word
I am ignorant	I am in a constant state of learning I am mindful of the Lord	• "For who has known the mind of the Lord that he may instruct him? But I have the mind of Christ." (NIV 1 Corinthians 2:16) • "You will keep in perfect peace I whose mind is steadfast, because I trust in you Lord." (NIV Isaiah 26:3) • "God will put his law in my mind and write it on my heart. He will be my God, and I am His son or daughter." (NIV Jeremiah 31:33)
I am irresponsible I am rebellious I am defiant I am disobedient I am stubborn	I am responsible I am submissive I am a slave to obedience... to Jesus Christ	• "As I am willing and obedient, I will eat the best from the land." (NIV Isaiah 1:19) • "I know that when I offer myself to someone to obey him as a slave, I am a slave to the one whom I obey—whether I am a slave to sin, which leads to death, or to obedience, which leads to righteousness."

Lie	Truth	Validated by God's Word
I am overbearing I am domineering I am dictatorial I am controlling	I am trusting I am submissive	• "And again, "I will put my trust in him." And again he says, "Here am I, and the children God has given me." (NIV Hebrews 2:13) • "The LORD is my strength and my shield; my heart trusts in him, and I am helped. My heart leaps for joy and I will give thanks to him in song." (NIV Psalm 28:7)
I am arrogant I am egotistical	I am modest I am humble I am reverent	• "Blessed are the meek, for they will inherit the earth." (NIV Matthew 5:5) • "God opposes the proud but gives grace to the humble. I humble myself, therefore, under God's mighty hand, that He may lift me up in due time." (NIV 1 Peter 5:6) • "I know that it will go better with God-fearing men, who are reverent before God." (NIV Ecclesiastes 8:12)

Lie	Truth	Validated by God's Word
I am hateful	I am loving I am kind I am gentle	• "And this is love: that I AM walking in obedience to his commands. As I have heard from the beginning, his command is that I walk in love." (NIV 2 John 1:6) • "I love my enemies and do good to them, and lend to them without expecting to get anything back. My reward will be great, and I am a son or daughter of the Most High, because He is kind to the ungrateful and wicked." (NIV Luke 6:35) • "My gentle answer turns away wrath, but a harsh word stirs up anger." (NIV Proverbs 15:1) • "I am taking His yoke upon me and learning from Him for He is gentle and humble in heart, and I am finding rest for my soul." (NIV Matthew 11:29)
I am a jerk magnet	I am a Godly man or woman magnet	• "Know that the LORD has set apart the Godly for himself; the LORD will hear when I call to Him." (Psalm 4:3)
I am a Man-izer or Woman-izer	I am respectful and honorable towards men and women	• "I love my wife, or girlfriend, just as Christ loved the church and gave Himself up for her to make her holy, cleansing her by the washing with water through the word, and to present her to himself as a radiant church, without stain or wrinkle or any other blemish, but holy and blameless." (NIV Ephesians 5:25-27) • "In this same way, I love my wife as my own body. And because I love my wife I love myself." (NIV Ephesians 5:28)

Lie	Truth	Validated by God's Word
I am promiscuous	I am committed to having sex only in marriage I am in control of my flesh I am morally sound	• "I am honoring the man or woman in my life, and my marriage bed is kept pure, for God will judge the adulterer and all the sexually immoral." (NIV Hebrews 13:4)
I am a drunk	I am sober I am drunk in the Spirit	• "I do not get drunk on wine, which leads to debauchery. Instead, I am filled with the Spirit." (NIV Ephesians 5:18) • "I am behaving decently, as in the daytime, not in orgies and drunkenness, not in sexual immorality and debauchery, not in dissension and jealousy. Rather, I am clothing myself with the Lord Jesus Christ, and I do not think about how to gratify the desires of my sinful nature." (NIV Romans 13:13-14)
I am resentful	I am forgiving I am gracious	• "I am bearing and forgiving whatever grievances I may have towards another. I forgive as the Lord forgives me. And over all these virtues I put on love, which binds them all together in perfect unity." (NIV Colossians 3:13-14) • "I forget the former things; and do not dwell on the past." (NIV Isaiah 43:18) • "Above all, I love others deeply, because love covers over a multitude of sins." (NIV 1 Peter 4:8)

Lie	Truth	Validated by God's Word
I am a procrastinator	I am a doer I am diligent I am responsible with my time	• "I am a doer of the word and not a hearer only." (KJV James 1:22) • "Whatever my hand finds to do, I do it with all my might, for in the grave, where I am going, there is neither working, nor planning, nor knowledge, nor wisdom." (NIV Ecclesiastes 9:10)
I am prideful	I am with humility I am humble	• "I am humble before the Lord, and He will lift me up." (NIV James 4:10) • "But He gives me more grace. That is why Scripture says: "God opposes the proud but gives grace to the humble." (NIV James 4:6)
I am alone	I am always in the presence of the Lord I am surrounded	• "I will fear not, for the Lord is with me and will bless me." (KJV Genesis 26:24)
I am unwanted I am undesirable	I am wanted I am favored I am treasured	• "'I have loved you,' says the LORD." (NIV Malachi 1:2) • "For surely, O LORD, you bless the righteous; you surround me with your favor as with a shield." (NIV Psalm 5:12) • "For I am a person holy to the LORD my God. Out of all the peoples on the face of the earth, the LORD has chosen me to be his treasured possession." (NIV Deuteronomy 14:2) • "You have stolen my heart, my sister, my bride; you have stolen my heart with one glance of your eyes, with one jewel of your necklace." (NIV Song of Solomon 4:9)

Lie	Truth	Validated by God's Word
I am lonely	I am known I am accepting of my status now I am willing to make new friends	• "Nevertheless, God's solid foundation stands firm, sealed with this inscription: 'The Lord knows me,' and I am confessing the name of the Lord and I must turn away from wickedness." (NIV 2 Timothy 2:19) • "'For I know the plans I have for you,' declares the LORD, 'plans to prosper you and not to harm you, plans to give you hope and a future.'" (NIV Jeremiah 29:11)
I am jealous	I am encouraging	• "But I encourage others daily, as long as it is called Today, so that I may not be hardened by sin's deceitfulness." (NIV Hebrews 3:13) • "Heal the sick, raise the dead, cleanse those who have leprosy, drive out demons. Freely I have received, freely I give." (NIV Matthew 10:8)
I am ashamed	I am forgiving of myself I am righteous I am pure	• "Everyone who has this hope in him purifies himself, just as he is pure." (NIV 1 John 3:3) • "The man and his wife were both naked, and they felt no shame." (NIV Genesis 2:25) • "I look to him and I am radiant; my face is never covered with shame." (NIV Psalm 34:5)

Lie	Truth	Validated by God's Word
I am hopeless	I am hopeful I am redeemed	• "But God will redeem my life from the grave; He will surely take me to Himself. Selah" (NIV Psalm 49:15) • "Find rest, O my soul, in God alone; my hope comes from him." (NIV Psalm 62:5) • "Not only so, but I also rejoice in my sufferings, because I know that suffering produces perseverance; perseverance, character; and character, hope. And hope does not disappoint me, because God has poured out his love into my heart by the Holy Spirit, whom He has given me." (NIV Romans 5:5) • "I have this hope as an anchor for my soul, firm and secure. It enters the inner sanctuary behind the curtain, where Jesus, who went before us, has entered on my behalf. He has become a high priest forever." (NIV Hebrews 6:19-20) • "Remember that I was a slave in Egypt and the LORD my God redeemed me." (NIV Deuteronomy 15:15)
I am unlovable	I am lovable I am treasured	• "He has taken me to the banquet hall, and His banner over me is love." (NIV Song of Solomon 2:4) • "Though the mountains be shaken and the hills be removed, yet God's unfailing love for me will not be shaken nor his covenant of peace be removed," says the LORD, who has compassion on me." (NIV Isaiah 54:10) • "This is how I know what love is: Jesus Christ laid down his life for me. And I ought to lay down my life for my brothers." (NIV 1 John 3:16)

Lie	Truth	Validated by God's Word
I am guilty **I am condemned**	**I am sanctified** **I am justified** **I am innocent**	• "Now I am committed to God and to the word of his grace, which can build me up and give me an inheritance among all those who are sanctified. " (Acts 20-32) • "For all have sinned and fall short of the glory of God, and are justified freely by his grace through the redemption that came by Christ Jesus." (Romans 3:23,24) • "Therefore, there is now no condemnation in me for I am in Christ Jesus, because through Christ Jesus the law of the Spirit of life set me free from the law of sin and death." (NIV Romans 8:1-2)
I am incapable	**I am capable** **I am powerful**	• "I am given the authority to trample on snakes and scorpions and to overcome all the power of the enemy; nothing will harm me." (NIV Luke 10:19) • "For God did not give me a spirit of timidity, but a spirit of power, of love and of self-discipline." (NIV 2 Timothy 1:7) • "I am putting on the full armor of God so that I can take my stand against the devil's schemes." (NIV Ephesians 6:11)

Lie	Truth	Validated by God's Word
I am weak I am tired	I am strong	• "May my Lord Jesus Christ Himself and God my Father, who loved me and by His grace gave me eternal encouragement and good hope, encourage my heart and strengthen me in every good deed and word." (NIV 2 Thessalonians 2:16-17)
	I am energetic	• "I am strong and courageous, not terrified or discouraged, for the LORD my God is with me wherever I go." (NIV Joshua 1:9)
	I am fired up	• "I can do all things through Christ who strengthens me." (NIV Philippians 4:13)
	I am enthusiastic	• "There remains, then, a Sabbath-rest for the people of God; for anyone who enters God's rest also rests from his own work, just as God did from his." (NIV Hebrews 4:9)
	I am rested	• "I am persevering so that when I have done the will of God, I will receive what He has promised." (NIV Hebrews 10:36)
I am too vulnerable	I am vulnerable I am open to love	• "For God did not give me a spirit of timidity, but a spirit of power, of love and of self-discipline." (NIV 2 Timothy 1:7)

Lie	Truth	Validated by God's Word
I am vengeful	I am giving I am kind	• "I am aware that vengeance is the Lord's; He will repay any harm done to me. I know the Lord will judge His people." (NIV Hebrews 10:30) • "I am the most excellent of men or women and my lips have been anointed with grace, since God has blessed me forever." (NIV Psalm 45:2) • "Let my conversation be always full of grace, seasoned with salt, so that I may know how to answer everyone." (NIV Colossians 4:6)
I am defeated	I am victorious I am more than a conqueror I am a winner	• "For in Christ all the fullness of the Deity lives in bodily form, and I am given fullness in Christ, who is the head over every power and authority." (NIV Colossians 2:9-10) • "No, in all these things I am more than a conqueror through Him who loves me." (NIV Romans 8:37) • "But thanks be to God! I am given the victory through my Lord Jesus Christ." (NIV 1 Corinthians 15:57) • "He will swallow up death in victory; and the Lord God will wipe away tears off my face; and the rebuke of His people shall he take away from off all the earth: for the Lord hath spoken it." (KJV Isaiah 25:8)

Lie	Truth	Validated by God's Word
I am inadequate	I am more than adequate I am powerful	• "For the kingdom of God is not a matter of talk but of power." (NIV 1 Corinthians 4:20) • "I have been given authority to trample on snakes and scorpions and to overcome all the power of the enemy; nothing will harm me." (NIV Luke 10:19)
I am rejected	I am chosen I am accepted	• "But I am a chosen person, a royal priesthood, a holy nation, a person belonging to God, that I may declare the praises of Him who called me out of darkness into His wonderful light." (NIV 1 Peter 2:9) • "How delightful is your love, my sister, my bride! How much more pleasing is your love than wine, and the fragrance of your perfume than any spice!" (NIV Song of Solomon 4:10)

Lie	Truth	Validated by God's Word
I am non-trusting of myself or others	I am trusting of others and of myself	• "I will have no fear of bad news; my heart is steadfast, trusting in the LORD." (NIV Psalm 112:7) • "But let me who takes refuge in you be glad; let me ever sing for joy. Spread Your protection over me, that I who love Your name may rejoice in You." (NIV Psalm 5:11) • "As for God, His way is perfect; the word of the LORD is flawless. He is a shield for me who takes refuge in Him." (NIV Psalm 18:30) • "I trust in the LORD with all my heart and lean not on my own understanding." (NIV Proverbs 3:5) • "In God I trust; I will not be afraid. What can man do to me?" (NIV Psalm 56:11)
I am a poor communicator	I am a good communicator I am communicative	• "For it will not be me speaking, but the Spirit of my Father speaking through me." (NIV Matthew 10:20) • "And these signs shall follow me; In Jesus name shall I cast out devils; I shall speak with new tongues." (KJV Mark 16:17) • "The Spirit gives life; the flesh counts for nothing. The words God have spoken to me are spirit and they are life." (NIV John 6:63)

Lie	Truth	Validated by God's Word
I am depressed	I am joyous I am motivated I am inspired I am enthusiastic	• "I have loved righteousness and hated wickedness; therefore God, my God, has set me above my companions by anointing me with the oil of joy." (NIV Hebrews 1:9) • "I have light, and gladness, and joy, and honor." (KJV Esther 8:16) • "But let me who takes refuge in You be glad; let me ever sing for joy. Spread Your protection over me, that I who love Your name may rejoice in You." (NIV Psalm 5:11) • "Restore to me the joy of your salvation and grant me a willing spirit, to sustain me." (NIV Psalm 51:12) • "To appoint unto me that mourn in Zion, to give unto me beauty for ashes, the oil of joy for mourning, the garment of praise for the spirit of heaviness; that I might be called a tree of righteousness, the planting of the Lord, that He might be glorified." (KJV Isaiah 61:3)

Lie	Truth	Validated by God's Word
I am just the way I am	I am forever changing into the likeness of Christ	• "He chose to give me birth through the word of truth, that I might be a kind of first-fruits of all he created." (NIV James 1:18) • "For I am predestined to be conformed to the likeness of His Son, that I might be the firstborn among many brothers or sisters. And those God predestined, he also called; those he called, He also justified; those He justified, He also glorified." (NIV Romans 8:29-30) • "Ask now about the former days, long before your time, from the day God created man on the earth; ask from one end of the heavens to the other. Has anything so great as this ever happened, or has anything like it ever been heard of?" (NIV Deuteronomy 4:32) • "For I am born again, not of perishable seed, but of imperishable, through the living and enduring word of God." (NIV 1 Peter 1:23) • "For I am God's workmanship, created in Christ Jesus to do good works, which God prepared in advance for me to do." (NIV Ephesians 2:10) • "For You created my inmost being; You knit me together in my mother's womb. I praise You because I am fearfully and wonderfully made; Your works are wonderful, I know that full well." (NIV Psalm 139:13-14)

Lie	Truth	Validated by God's Word
I am a bad husband or wife	**I am a holy husband or holy wife**	<ul><li>"I am a wife of noble character and am my husband's crown," (NIV Proverbs 12:4)</li><li>"I am a good husband and render unto my wife due benevolence." (KJV 1 Corinthians 7:3)</li><li>"I am a good wife and render unto my husband due benevolence." (KJV 1 Corinthians 7:3)</li><li>"For my husband is the head of me, even as Christ is the head of the church: and he is the saviour of the body." (KJV Ephesians 5:23)</li><li>"For I am the head of my wife, even as Christ is the head of the church: and I am the saviour of the body." (KJV Ephesians 5:23)</li><li>**Remember:** This refers to the husband as the spiritual head of the family. He is to lead his family with the love and gentleness and protection of Jesus Christ and is to lay down his life for his family as Jesus did for us. It doesn't at all imply ruler, dictator, boss, or punisher. Women, it is up to you to choose a man *worthy* of submitting to, someone willing to lay down his life for you!</li></ul>

Lie	Truth	Validated by God's Word
I am a bad son or daughter	I am a good son or daughter I am a child of God	• "I am doing everything without complaining, or arguing, so that I may become blameless and pure, a child of God without fault in a crooked and depraved generation, in which I shine like stars in the universe." (NIV Philippians 2:14-15) • "I have received Him, and I believe in Him, and I have been given the right to be called a child of God." (NIV John 1:12) • "The Spirit Himself testifies with our spirit that we are God's children." (NIV Romans 8:16)
I am a bad friend	I am a good friend	• "I am loving my friends at all times, and I was born for adversity." (NIV Proverbs 17:17) • "Perfume and incense bring joy to the heart, and the pleasantness of my friend springs from his or her earnest counsel." (NIV Proverbs 27:9) • "As iron sharpens iron, so one man sharpens another." (NIV Proverbs 27:17)

Lie	Truth	Validated by God's Word
I am poor at managing my money	I am a good steward of God's gifts	• "Come, all you who are thirsty, come to the waters; and you who have no money, come, buy and eat! Come, buy wine and milk without money and without cost. Why spend money on what is not bread, and your labor on what does not satisfy? Listen, listen to me, and eat what is good, and your soul will delight in the richest of fare." (NIV Isaiah 15:22) • "The Lord answered, 'Who then is the faithful and wise manager, whom the master puts in charge of his servants to give them their food allowance at the proper time?' " (NIV Luke 12:42)
I am unhealthy I am unwilling to eat healthy food	I am healthy I am willing to eat healthy food	• "There is a way that seems right to me, but in the end it leads to death." (NIV Proverbs 16:25) • "I know my body is a temple of the Holy Spirit, who is in me, whom I have received from God; I am not my own; I was bought at a price—therefore I will honor God with my body." (NIV 1 Corinthians 6:19-20)
I am not as young as I used to be I am old	I am exactly where God wants me to be	• "The glory of young men is their strength, gray hair the splendor of the old." (NIV Proverbs 20:29) • "And afterward, I will pour out my Spirit on all people. Your sons and daughters will prophesy, your old men will dream dreams, your young men will see visions." (NIV Joel 2:28) • "Is not wisdom found among the aged? Does not long life bring understanding?" (NIV Job 12:12)

Lie	Truth	Validated by God's Word
I am not a leader	I am a leader	• "You have delivered me from the attacks of the people; you have made me the head of nations; people I did not know are subject to me." (NIV Psalm 18:43) • "And I have been given fullness in Christ, who is the head over every power and authority." (NIV Colossians 2:10)
I am impatient	I am patient	• "Love is patient, love is kind. It does not envy, it does not boast, it is not proud." (NIV 1 Corinthians 13:4) • "For whatsoever things were written aforetime were written for our learning, that we through patience and comfort of the scriptures might have hope. Now the God of patience and consolation grant you to be likeminded one toward another according to Christ Jesus." (KJV Romans 15:4) • "Be completely humble and gentle; be patient, bearing with one another in love." (NIV Ephesians 4:2)
I am judgmental	I am understanding I am compassionate	• "Be kind and compassionate to one another, forgiving each other, just as in Christ God forgave you." (Ephesians 4:32) • "But it is the spirit in me, the breath of the Almighty, that gives me understanding." (NIV Job 32:8) • "Discretion will protect me, and understanding will guard me." (NIV Proverbs 2:11)

Lie	Truth	Validated by God's Word
I am stubborn	I am willing	• "Wash away all my iniquity and cleanse me from my sin." (NIV Psalm 51:2) • "Therefore, since Christ suffered in his body, arm yourselves also with the same attitude, because he who has suffered in his body is done with sin." (NIV 1 Peter 4:1)
I am immature	I am learning I am growing in the Lord	• "Men will dwell again in his shade. He will flourish like the grain. He will blossom like a vine, and his fame will be like the wine from Lebanon." (NIV Hosea 14:7) • "But for myself who reveres God's name, the son of righteousness will rise with healing in its wings. And I will go out and leap like calves released from the stall." (NIV Malachi 4:2) • "Let the wise listen and add to their learning, and let the discerning get guidance." (NIV Proverbs 1:5) • "For everything that was written in the past was written to teach me, so that through endurance and the encouragement of the Scriptures I might have hope." (NIV Romans 15:4)
I am confused	I am confident	• "The law of the LORD is perfect, reviving the soul. The statutes of the LORD are trustworthy, making wise the simple." (NIV Psalm 19:7) • "In you, O LORD, I have taken refuge; let me never be put to shame." (NIV Psalm 71:1) • "For God is not a God of disorder but of peace." (NIV 1 Corinthians 14:33)

Lie	Truth	Validated by God's Word
I am doubtful	I am sure I am positive	• "The law of the LORD is perfect, reviving the soul. The statutes of the LORD are trustworthy, making wise the simple." (NIV Psalm 19:7) • "We believe and know that you are the Holy One of God." (NIV John 6:69) • "Nevertheless, God's solid foundation stands firm, sealed with this inscription: 'The Lord knows me because I am His,' and, 'I am confessing the name of the Lord and must turn away from wickedness.' " (NIV 2 Timothy 2:19)
I am deceptive	I am truthful	• "Truthful lips endure forever, but a lying tongue lasts only a moment." (NIV Proverbs 12:19) • "Faithfulness springs forth from the earth, and righteousness looks down from heaven." (NIV Psalm 85:11) • "My mouth speaks what is true, for my lips detest wickedness." (NIV Proverbs 8:7)

Lie	Truth	Validated by God's Word
I am compromising	I am faithful	• "A wicked messenger falls into trouble, but a trustworthy envoy brings healing." (NIV Proverbs 13:17) • "His master replied, 'Well done, good and faithful servant! You have been faithful with a few things; I will put you in charge of many things. Come and share your master's happiness!' " (NIV Matthew 25:21) • "Let me hold unswervingly to the hope I profess, for he who promised is faithful." (NIV Hebrews 10:23) • "They will make war against the Lamb, but the Lamb will overcome them because he is Lord of lords and King of kings—and with Him will be His called, chosen and faithful followers." (NIV Revelation 17:14)
I am racist I am prejudice	I am a lover of all people	• "A new command I give you: love one another. As I have loved you, so you must love one another." (John 13:34) • "You, my brothers, were called to be free. But do not use your freedom to indulge the sinful nature; rather, serve one another in love." (NIV Galatians 5:13)
I am insecure	I am secure	• "I am living in a peaceful dwelling place, in a secure home, in undisturbed places of rest." (NIV Isaiah 32:18) • "I am confident of this, that he who began a good work in me will carry it on to completion until the day of Christ Jesus." (Philippians 1:6) • "Should not my piety be your confidence and your blameless ways your hope?" (NIV Job 4:6) • "I have come to share in Christ if I hold firmly till the end the confidence I had at first." (NIV Hebrews 3:14)

Lie	Truth	Validated by God's Word
I am divorced	I am single I am in covenant with the Lord	• "I now establish my covenant with you and with your descendants after you." (NIV Genesis 9:9) • "I will not violate my covenant or alter what my lips have uttered." (NIV Psalm 89:34) • "This is the covenant I will make with the house of Israel after that time, declares the Lord. God will put His laws in my mind and write them on my heart. He will be my God, and we will be His people." (NIV Hebrews 8:10) • "For your Maker is your husband—the LORD Almighty is his name—the Holy One of Israel is your Redeemer; he is called the God of all the earth." (NIV Isaiah 54:5)
I am too emotional I am too sensitive	I am stable	• "A friend loves at all times, and a brother is born for adversity." (NIV Proverbs 17:17) • "A quick-tempered man does foolish things, and a crafty man is hated." (NIV Proverbs 14:17)

Lie	Truth	Validated by God's Word
I am suspicious	I am trusting	• "I will have no fear of bad news; my heart is steadfast, trusting in the LORD." (NIV Psalm 112:7) • "But I, who take refuge in you, am glad; let me ever sing for joy. Spread your protection over me, that I, who love your name, may rejoice in you." (NIV Psalm 5:11) • "As for God, his way is perfect; the word of the LORD is flawless. He is a shield for all who take refuge in him." (NIV Psalm 18:30) • "I am trusting in the LORD with all my heart and leaning not on my own understanding." (NIV Proverbs 3:5) • "In God I trust; I will not be afraid. What can man do to me?" (NIV Psalm 56:11)
I am too competitive	I am content	• "I know what it is to be in need, and I know what it is to have plenty. I have learned the secret of being content in any and every situation, whether well fed or hungry, whether living in plenty or in want." (NIV Philippians 4:12) • "I am keeping my life free from the love of money and being content with what I have, because God has said, 'Never will I leave you; never will I forsake you.'" (NIV Hebrews 13:5) • "May the God of hope fill me with all joy and peace as I trust in him, so that I may overflow with hope by the power of the Holy Spirit." (NIV Romans 15:13)

Lie	Truth	Validated by God's Word
I am insensitive	I am sensitive, understanding, gentle	• "And I am full with the Spirit of God, with skill, ability and knowledge in all kinds of crafts." (NIV Exodus 31:3) • "For the kingdom of God is not a matter of talk but of power." (NIV 1 Corinthians 4:20) • "But the wisdom that comes from heaven is first of all pure; then peace-loving, considerate, submissive, full of mercy and good fruit, impartial and sincere." (NIV James 3:17)
I am too trusting	I am trusting	• "Those who know your name will trust in you, for you, LORD, have never forsaken those who seek you." (NIV Psalm 9:10) • "As for God, his way is perfect; the word of the LORD is flawless. He is a shield for me who takes refuge in him." (NIV Psalm 18:30) • "I am trusting in the Lord with all my heart and I am not leaning on my own understanding." (NIV Proverbs 3:5)

Lie	Truth	Validated by God's Word
I am a hypocrite	I am a doer of the Word I am loving I am a believer	• "But as I look intently into the perfect law that gives freedom, and continue to do this, not forgetting what I have heard, but doing it—I am blessed in what I do." (NIV James 1:25) • "With his mouth the godless destroys his neighbor, but through knowledge the righteous." (NIV Proverbs 11:9) • "Teach me knowledge and good judgment, for I believe in your commands." (NIV Proverbs 119:66) • "'If you can?' said Jesus. 'Everything is possible for him who believes.'" (NIV Mark 9:23) • "And without faith it is impossible to please God, because anyone who comes to him must believe that he exists and that he rewards those who earnestly seek him." (Hebrews 11:6)
I am a liar and cheater	I am honest	• "But when he, the Spirit of truth, comes, he will guide me into all truth. He will not speak on his own; he will speak only what he hears, and he will tell me what is yet to come." (NIV John 16:13) • "I am speaking the truth in Christ—I am not lying, my conscience confirms it in the Holy Spirit." (NIV Romans 9:1) • "Surely you desire truth in the inner parts; you teach me wisdom in the inmost place." (Psalm 51:6) • "My mouth speaks what is true, for my lips detest wickedness." (Proverbs 8:7)

Lie	Truth	Validated by God's Word
I am humiliated	**I am confident**	• "This is what the Sovereign LORD, the Holy One of Israel, says: "In repentance and rest is your salvation, in quietness and trust is your strength, but you would have none of it." (NIV Isaiah 30:15) • "The LORD is my strength and my song; he has become my salvation. He is my God, and I will praise him, my father's God, and I will exalt him." (NIV Exodus 15:2) • "I love the LORD my God with all my heart and with all my soul and with all your strength." (NIV Deuteronomy 6:5)
I am sad	**I am glad**	• "I am happy. Let me sing songs of praise." (James 5:13) • "Therefore my heart is glad and my tongue rejoices; my body also will rest secure." (NIV Psalm 16:9) • "For you make me glad by your deeds, O LORD ; I sing for joy at the works of your hands." (NIV Psalm 92:4) • "And the ransomed of the LORD will return. I will enter Zion with singing; everlasting joy will crown my head. Gladness and joy will overtake me, and sorrow and sighing will flee away." (NIV Isaiah 35:10)

Lie	Truth	Validated by God's Word
I am sorrowful	I am joyful	• "Then my soul will rejoice in the LORD and delight in his salvation." (NIV Psalm 35:9) • "These I will bring to my holy mountain and give them joy in my house of prayer. Their burnt offerings and sacrifices will be accepted on my altar; for my house will be called a house of prayer for all nations." (NIV Isaiah 56:7) • "The ransomed of the LORD will return. They will enter Zion with singing; everlasting joy will crown their heads. Gladness and joy will overtake them, and sorrow and sighing will flee away." (NIV Isaiah 51:11)
I am suicidal	I am a lover of life	• "How much more, then, will the blood of Christ, who through the eternal Spirit offered himself unblemished to God, cleanse my conscience from acts that lead to death, so that I may serve the living God!" (NIV Hebrews 9:14) • "I will not die but live, and will proclaim what the LORD has done." (NIV Psalm 118:17) • "Sustain me according to your promise, and I will live; do not let my hopes be dashed." (NIV Psalm 119:116)

Lie	Truth	Validated by God's Word
I am a homosexual	I am a heterosexual I am pure I am holy	• "I honor a marriage between a man and a woman, and my marriage bed kept pure, for God will judge the adulterer and all the sexually immoral." (NIV Hebrews 13:4) "You say to God, 'My beliefs are flawless and I am pure in your sight.' " (NIV Job 11:4) • "Cleanse me with hyssop, and I will be clean; wash me, and I will be whiter than snow." (NIV Psalm 51:7) • "You are already clean because of the word I have spoken to you." (NIV John 15:3)
I am unreasonable	I am reasonable I am wise	• "Let the wise listen and add to their learning, and let the discerning get guidance." (NIV Proverbs 1:5) • "Words from a wise man's mouth are gracious, but a fool is consumed by his own lips." (NIV Ecclesiastes 10:12) • "He changes times and seasons; he sets up kings and deposes them. He gives wisdom to the wise and knowledge to the discerning." (NIV Daniel 2:21) • "My mouth will speak words of wisdom; the utterance from my heart will give understanding." (NIV Psalm 49:3)

Lie	Truth	Validated by God's Word
I am cranky	I am happy	• "You have made known to me the path of life; you will fill me with joy in your presence, with eternal pleasures at your right hand." (NIV Psalm 16:11) • "But let me, who takes refuge in you, be glad; let me ever sing for joy. Spread your protection over me, that I, who loves your name, may rejoice in you." (NIV Psalm 5:11) • "Blessed are you, O Israel! Who is like you, a people saved by the LORD? He is my shield and helper and my glorious sword. My enemies will cower before you, and you will trample down their high places." (NIV Deuteronomy 3:29)
I am vain	I am humble I am meek	• "Blessed are the meek, for they will inherit the earth." (NIV Matthew 5:5) • "Now my eyes will be open and my ears attentive to the prayers offered in this place." (NIV 2 Chronicles 7:15) • "But I will leave within you the meek and humble, who trust in the name of the LORD." (NIV Zephaniah 3:12) • "For the LORD takes delight in me; he crowns the humble with salvation." (NIV Psalm 149:4)

Lie	Truth	Validated by God's Word
I am superior	I am modest I am humble before the Lord	• "Pride goes before destruction, a haughty spirit before a fall." (NIV Proverbs 16:18) • "The LORD takes delight in me; he crowns the humble with salvation." (Psalm 149:4) • "If my people, who are called by my name, will humble themselves and pray and seek my face and turn from their wicked ways, then will I hear from heaven and will forgive their sin and will heal their land." (2 Chronicles 7:14)
I am independent	I am dependent only on God	• "My salvation and my honor depend on God; he is my mighty rock, my refuge." (Psalm 62:7) • "Who among you fears the LORD and obeys the word of his servant? Let him who walks in the dark, who has no light, trust in the name of the LORD and rely on his God." (Isaiah 50:10) • "And so I know and rely on the love God has for me. God is love. Whoever lives in love lives in God, and God in him." (NIV 1 John 4:16)

Lie	Truth	Validated by God's Word
I am self-righteous	I am righteous through the blood of Jesus	• "What is more, I consider everything a loss compared to the surpassing greatness of knowing Christ Jesus my Lord, for whose sake I have lost all things. I consider them rubbish, that I may gain Christ and be found in him, not having a righteousness of my own that comes from the law, but that which is through faith in Christ—the righteousness that comes from God and is by faith." (NIV Philippians 3:8-9) • "My tongue will speak of your righteousness and of your praises all day long." (NIV Psalm 35:28) • "I walk in the way of righteousness, along the paths of justice." (NIV Proverbs 8:20)
I am rude	I am gracious	• "The LORD is compassionate and gracious, slow to anger, abounding in love." (NIV Psalm 103:8) • "Words from a wise man's mouth are gracious, but a fool is consumed by his own lips." (NIV Ecclesiastes 10:12)
I am seductive	I am innocent I am virtuous	• "And now, my daughter, don't be afraid. I will do for you all you ask. All my fellow townsmen know that you are a woman of noble character." (NIV Ruth 3:11) • "A wife of noble character who can find? She is worth far more than rubies." (Proverbs 31:10) • "I am blameless and pure, a child of God without fault in a crooked and depraved generation, in which I shine like stars in the universe." (NIV Philippians 2:15)

Lie	Truth	Validated by God's Word
I am open to everything	I am committed	• "I commit to the LORD whatever I do, and my plans will succeed." (NIV Proverbs 16:3) • "Therefore, I stand firm. Let nothing move me. I always give myself fully to the work of the Lord, because I know that my labor in the Lord is not in vain." (NIV 1 Corinthians 15:58)
I am afraid of death and dying	I am a lover of life	• "For you have delivered me from death and my feet from stumbling, that I may walk before God in the light of life."(NIV Psalm 56:13) • "He is not the God of the dead, but of the living, for to him all are alive." (NIV Luke 20:38) • "Jesus said to her, 'I am the resurrection and the life. He who believes in me will live, even though he dies.'" (John 11:25)
I am unfruitful	I am fruitful	• "You did not choose me, but I chose you and appointed you to go and bear fruit—fruit that will last. Then the Father will give you whatever you ask in my name." (NIV John 15:16) • "I will make you very fruitful; I will make nations of you, and kings will come from you." (NIV Genesis 17:6) • "I myself will gather the remnant of my flock out of all the countries where I have driven them and will bring them back to their pasture, where they will be fruitful and increase in number." (NIV Jeremiah 23:3)

Lie	Truth	Validated by God's Word
I am unfaithful	I am faithful	• "Know therefore that the LORD your God is Good; he is the faithful God, keeping his covenant of love to a thousand generations of those who love him and keep his commands." (NIV Deuteronomy 7:9) • "God, who has called me into fellowship with his Son Jesus Christ our Lord, is faithful." (NIV 1 Colossians 1:9) • "If I am faithless, he will remain faithful, for he cannot disown himself." (NIV 2 Timothy 2:13) • "They will make war against the Lamb, but the Lamb will overcome them because he is Lord of lords and King of kings—and with him will be his called, chosen and faithful followers." (NIV Revelation 17:14)
I am too critical	I am accepting I am loving	• "A new command I give you: Love one another. As I have loved you, so you must love one another." (NIV John 13:34)
I am stressed	I am calm	• "I am not anxious about anything, but in everything, by prayer and petition, with thanksgiving, I present my requests to God." (NIV Philippians 4:6) • "My people will live in peaceful dwelling places, in secure homes, in undisturbed places of rest." (NIV Isaiah 32:18) • "The LORD my God is with me, he is mighty to save. He will take great delight in me, he will quiet me with his love, he will rejoice over me with singing." (NIV Zephaniah 3:17)

Lie	Truth	Validated by God's Word
I am afraid to fail	I am open to failure, yet in Jesus I am victorious!	• "I will not have to fight this battle. I take up my position; standing firm and see the deliverance the LORD will give me, O Judah and Jerusalem. Do not be afraid; do not be discouraged. Go out to face them tomorrow, and the LORD will be with you." (NIV 2 Chronicles 20:17) • "The LORD will guide me always; he will satisfy my needs in a sun-scorched land and will strengthen my frame. I will be like a well-watered garden, like a spring whose waters never fail." (NIV Isaiah 58:11)
I am afraid to succeed	I am excited to walk in victory!	• "They gave toward the work on the temple of God five thousand talents and ten thousand darics of gold, ten thousand talents of silver, eighteen thousand talents of bronze and a hundred thousand talents of iron." (NIV 1 Chronicles 29:7) • "For everyone born of God overcomes the world. This is the victory that has overcome the world, even our faith." (NIV 1 John 5:4)

Lie	Truth	Validated by God's Word
I am cursed	I am blessed	• "All these blessings will come upon me and accompany me if I obey the LORD my God: I will be blessed in the city and blessed in the country. The fruit of my womb will be blessed, and the crops of my land and the young of my livestock-the calves of my herds and the lambs of my flocks. My basket and my kneading trough will be blessed. I will be blessed when I come in and blessed when I go out." (NIV Deuteronomy 28:2-6) • "Then the King will say to those on his right, 'Come, you who are blessed by my Father; take your inheritance, the kingdom prepared for you since the creation of the world.'" (NIV Matthew 25:34) • "Blessed are the poor in spirit, for theirs is the kingdom of heaven." (NIV Matthew 5:3)
I am a poor listener	I am a good listener	• "Listen, for I have worthy things to say; I open my lips to speak what is right." (NIV Proverbs 4:6) • "Let me hear joy and gladness; let the bones you have crushed rejoice." (NIV Psalm 51:8) • "He who has ears, let him hear." (NIV Matthew 11:15) • "But blessed are your eyes because they see, and your ears because they hear." (NIV Matthew 13:16)

Lie	Truth	Validated by God's Word
I am too giving	**I am giving**	• "Be devoted to one another in brotherly love. Honor one another above yourselves." (Romans 12:10) • "I am giving what I have decided in my heart to give, not reluctantly or under compulsion, for God loves a cheerful giver." (NIV 2 Corinthians 9:7) • "My mouth will speak words of wisdom; the utterance from my heart will give understanding." (NIV Psalm 49:3)
I am co-dependent	**I am dependent only on Jesus**	• "Who among you fears the LORD and obeys the word of his servant? Let him who walks in the dark, who has no light, trust in the name of the LORD and rely on his God." (NIV Isaiah 50:10) • "Yet I am poor and needy; may the Lord think of me. You are my help and my deliverer; O my God, do not delay." (Psalm 40:17) • "I am not saying this because I am in need, for I have learned to be content whatever the circumstances." (NIV Philippians 4:11) • "And my God will meet all my needs according to his glorious riches in Christ Jesus." (Philippians 4:19)
I am lustful	**I am innocent** **I am holy**	• "I am living by the Spirit, and I will not gratify the desires of my sinful nature." (NIV Galatians 5:16) • "You are to be holy to me because I, the LORD , am holy, and I have set you apart from the nations to be my own." (NIV Leviticus 20:26)

83

Lie	Truth	Validated by God's Word
I am a God	I am a man or woman saved through grace	• "I tell you that in the same way there will be more rejoicing in heaven over one sinner who repents than over ninety nine righteous persons who do not need to repent." (NIV Luke 15:17) • "But God demonstrates his own love for us in this: While we were still sinners, Christ died for us." (NIV Romans 5:8) • "For it is by grace I have been saved, through faith—and this not from yourselves, it is the gift of God." (NIV Ephesians 2:8)
I am sick	I am healthy	• "A cheerful look brings joy to the heart, and good news gives health to the bones." (NIV Proverbs 15:30) • "But I will restore you to health and heal your wounds,' declares the LORD , 'because you are called an outcast, Zion for whom no one cares." (NIV Jeremiah 30:17) • "Hope deferred makes the heart sick, but a longing fulfilled is a tree of life." (Proverbs 13:12) • "I will search for the lost and bring back the strays. I will bind up the injured and strengthen the weak, but the sleek and the strong I will destroy. I will shepherd the flock with justice." (NIV Ezekiel 34:16)

Lie	Truth	Validated by God's Word
I am wicked	I am innocent	• "'I am pure and without sin; I am clean and free from guilt." (NIV Job 33:9) • "Keep your servant also from willful sins; may they not rule over me. Then will I be blameless, innocent of great transgression." (NIV Psalm 19:13) • "I wash my hands in innocence, and go about your altar, O LORD." (NIV Psalm 26:6)
I am self-sabotaging	I am taking care of the gifts God has given me	• "Then the LORD said to Aaron, "I myself have put you in charge of the offerings presented to me; all the holy offerings the Israelites give me I give to you and your sons as your portion." (NIV Numbers 18:8) • "If you, then, though you are evil, know how to give good gifts to your children, how much more will your Father in heaven give good gifts to those who ask him!" (NIV Matthew 7:11) • "For God's gifts and his call are irrevocable." (NIV Romans 11:29)
I am passive	I am full of energy I am passionate	• "To this end I labor, struggling with all his energy, which so powerfully works in me." (NIV Colossians 1:29) • "For God did not give us a spirit of timidity, but a spirit of power, of love and self-discipline." (2 Timothy 1:7)

Lie	Truth	Validated by God's Word
I am a quitter	I am full of perseverance	• "Since you have kept my command to endure patiently, I will also keep you from the hour of trial that is going to come upon the whole world to test those who live on the earth." (NIV Revelation 3:10) • "As you know, we consider blessed those who have persevered. You have heard of Job's perseverance and have seen what the Lord finally brought about. The Lord is full of compassion and mercy." (NIV James 5:11) • "Not only so, but we also rejoice in our sufferings, because we know that suffering produces perseverance; perseverance, character; and character, hope." (Romans 5:3-4) • "For his anger lasts only a moment, but his favor lasts a lifetime; weeping may remain for a night, but rejoicing comes in the morning." (Psalm 30:5)
I am addicted to position or success	I am humble	• "I live in harmony with one another. I am not proud and I am willing to associate with people of low position. Do not be conceited" (NIV Romans 12:16) • "For the LORD takes delight in his people; he crowns the humble with salvation." (NIV Psalm 149:4) • "Take my yoke upon you and learn from me, for I am gentle and humble in heart, and you will find rest for your souls." (NIV Matthew 11:29)

Lie	Truth	Validated by God's Word
I am addicted to cigarettes or other drugs	**I am taking care of my body**	• "I have set the LORD always before me. Because he is at my right hand, I will not be shaken. Therefore my heart is glad and my tongue rejoices; my body also will rest secure, because you will not abandon me to the grave, nor will you let your Holy One see decay." (NIV Psalm 16:8-10) • "Do not offer the parts of your body to sin, as instruments of wickedness, but rather offer yourselves to God, as those who have been brought from death to life; and offer the parts of your body to him as instruments of righteousness." (NIV Romans 6:13) • "Do you not know that your body is a temple of the Holy Spirit, who is in you, whom you have received from God? You are not your own; you were bought at a price. Therefore honor God with your body." (NIV 1 Corinthians 6:19-20)
I am a complainer	**I am positive** **I am optimistic**	• "Do everything without complaining or arguing, so that you may become blameless and pure, children of God without fault in a crooked and depraved generation, in which you shine like stars in the universe." (NIV Philippians 4:14,15) • "Your attitude should be the same as that of Christ Jesus." (Philippians 2:5)

For Reflection:

In the spaces below, write down (in your own words) who Christ says you are.

_____

_____

Think back over the last week. Identify a negative thought or bad attitude you had and describe what effect it had on you.

_____

_____

This week (and every week), catch yourself in the act of entertaining a negative thought, or bad attitude, and stop the devil in his tracks. Immediately, affirm God's truth about the situation or event. Use the I AM chart to guide you into the truth.

_____

_____

_____

COMMITMENT & FORGIVENESS

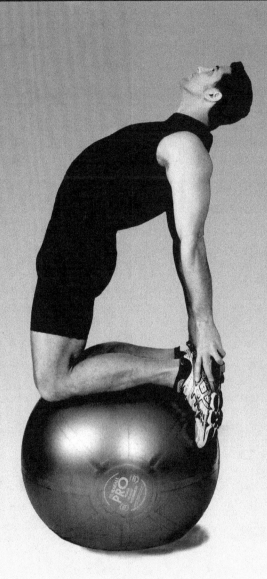

"But your hearts must be fully committed to the LORD our God, to live by his decrees and obey his commands, as at this time." (1 Kings 8:61)
"Bear with each other and forgive whatever grievances you may have against one another. Forgive as the Lord forgave you. And over all these virtues put on love, which binds them all together in perfect unity." (Colossians 3:13-14)

WEEK TWO

Ask Principle

Accountability . . . Support . . . Knowledge

Here we are in week 2 already! While reflecting on your life and your relationship with God this week, you will learn to **ASK** Him questions throughout your day. **"ASK and it will be given to you; seek and you will find; knock and the door will be opened to you. For everyone who asks receives; he who seeks finds; and to him who knocks, the door will be opened"** (Matthew 7:7–8). Every time you ASK God a question, His answers show up in one of these three categories: *a*ccountability, *s*upport, and *k*nowledge (the ASK principle).

*A*ccountability

Living in freedom as you make healthy lifestyle changes means being **"response-able"** and **"account-able"** with your decisions. But before I go further into why you need accountability and why it is so significant in your life, you need to be set free from the *legalistic repercussions of perfectionism*. Otherwise, accountability to and from others will hold you in the same bondage as the unhealthy lifestyle itself! If you (a) expect others to be perfect, or (b) others expect you to be perfect, or (c) both, you are in fact out of the will of God. Trying to be perfect defeats the very reason Christ died for each and every one of us. Perfectionism will control you and stress you out to the point of altogether breaking your commitment to be healthy.

I learned this principle the hard way—as I usually do. As a college student, I was teaching water skiing at a sports camp called Camp Caribou in Maine. One day the 7-time US barefoot water skiing champion Zenon Bilas came to the camp to give a demonstration, a flying dock start off a 10-foot lifeguard stand. This is where Zenon, while barefoot, jumps off a 10-foot high life guard stand while holding on to a ski rope that is connected to a competition ski boat. The powerful ski boat accelerates quickly and once Zenon hits the water he is yanked up and out of the water and water skis on his bare feet. Before the event, the other ski instructors and I went out with Zenon to learn to barefoot water ski. When my turn came, I mastered the boom, the short rope, and the foot-long skis on the long rope. Every time I got up and tried to barefoot on the long rope, I wiped out—time after time after time. I was becoming agitated. I hit the water a couple of times and yelled at myself to get more focused. I was very determined and put a lot of pressure on myself to succeed. When the boat came back around, Zenon met me with a stern look and said to me, "Brian, you are never going to get up with that attitude." *"Excuse me!"* I thought. *"What did you say?"* I was completely offended, of course. Inside I was saying, "Are you talking to me? Are *you* talking to *me?*" I thought I was doing a great job of keeping myself motivated and was determined not to give up. What he said next changed many things in my life . . . *again.*

Zenon told me to do *exactly* what he said and he wanted me to fall doing it. "You want me to do what?!" I said. And he repeated it. "I want you to do exactly what I say, and I want you to fall doing it." So I got behind the boat, disgusted at both myself and Zenon for telling me my attitude was bad and thought about what he said to me. While mumbling under my breath, I focused on exactly what he said to do with correct form and knew I needed to fall while doing it. This went against everything I was, everything I stood for! Brian Wellbrock does *not* fall on purpose! He is the one who scores the touchdowns, hits the homeruns, and demands perfection from himself. So what do you think happened? To my amazement, I popped up out of the water and barefoot water-skied for 20 seconds. It was exhilarating! You see, Zenon gave me permission to fail, so my focus was no longer on "not failing", but on doing what he said to do. The pressure I put on myself to succeed was lifted so I could simply focus on what I needed to do. The rest of the summer, I used this same teaching technique with all my kids, and the rate at which they learned was exponential. That was the beginning of my own freedom from perfectionism.

Remember this: If you want to succeed at anything, you must allow yourself to fail. I am not encouraging you to fail, but, I am telling you the truth—because of Jesus Christ, you have permission to fail. **Allowing yourself to fail, or acknowledging that you will at times, frees you from the burden of the perfection of success.** Why do you think Jesus did what He did for us? Here's why—because we are imperfect beings incapable of perfection. **"For all have sinned and fall short of the glory of God, and are justified freely by his grace through the redemption that came by Christ Jesus"** (Romans 3:23–24). Many of you have already failed with your health many times. That's OK. By the grace of Jesus Christ you are free to put those failures behind you.

Free and Accountable in Grace and Love

While you may be free from the perfection mentioned above, you still need to understand the importance of accountability. Accountability is not intended to condemn you but only to expose your difficulties so, that through humility and confession, you can receive the grace of Jesus Christ. **"Now we know that whatever the law says, it says to those who are under the law, so that every mouth may be silenced and the whole world be held accountable to God"** (Romans 3:19). This simply means that if you are overweight and out of shape and not living a healthy lifestyle, no problem. Stand up tall and admit your struggles and use the grace of God to propel you into a healthy lifestyle. Don't allow the law of taking care of yourself to be a burden—allow it to be a measure of your accountability.

"Account-ability" comes from being in relationships with other Christians in which you can give and receive encouragement and expose obedience and disobedience to God. Accountability comes from love and understanding, not from judgment, or ridicule. As Christ's followers, we are accountable to everyone in the form of either giving or receiving love. Jesus set the bar and we are to live as He would. He *is* inside of you after all. As you journal, notice how God answers many of your questions in the form of giving or receiving accountability to and from others. I encourage all of you to get involved in small groups or Bible studies in your church or community. Join one or start your own and together use the principles in this book and *Life Application Journal*. Be accountable to and for your friends and family, be free and love one another.

Two Stories of Accountability

To close this section on accountability, I will share two stories. I struggled for quite some time over whether to include these stories because I didn't want them to come across negative. In my heart, though, I felt God saying that this is the brutal reality of how important being healthy is. While training myself in Irving, Texas, I was doing a set of leg extensions by a window overlooking the parking lot and street. Something across the street caught my attention. A little boy no older that two or three was screaming and running at top speed straight toward the street. A ways back I saw a young woman who weighed approximately 350 pounds trying to make her way toward the little boy. The woman's face was dark and worn out and she looked as if she had just given up. She could barely move. It was clear to me that the little boy was going to beat her to the street. Just a few feet from the street, the boy turned down the sidewalk and kept running, this time toward a six-lane street and four-way intersection. My heart was pounding. By this time I was out in the parking lot ready to sprint across the street when I saw the young woman muster every ounce of energy she could to run toward the little boy. Still, I could see that she wasn't going to make it in time. She simply could not move fast enough. I prayed as I ran toward him. At that instant, just as the boy was about to hurtle into the oncoming traffic, he ducked instead behind one of those big green traffic light boxes on the corner of the intersection. The young woman finally reached him and was so exhausted that she had to practically lie on him to calm him down. Besides the grace of God and possibly a quick prayer, I don't know what made him stop and decide to hide instead of continue to run into the street. My heart races even now as I remember seeing the boy stop just before he ran into the street.

So why would I write this in a section on accountability? That woman was accountable to that little boy. She wasn't just accountable *for* him, but *to* him. She was the adult, and it was her responsibility as his protector to, in fact, protect him, even from himself. Bottom line is that your health is as important as anything you have. Had this little boy been hit by a car, in my opinion, it would have been because of the young woman's negligence. After witnessing this event, it took hours for my heart to slow down. We do not exercise merely to honor God or to gain self-esteem, but to save lives like that little boy's. I am not only accountable within my adult relationships. I am not solely responsible, or *accountable for* my children. I am *accountable to them* to take care of myself as their provider, protector, and caretaker. Do you see the difference? Perhaps you are reading this right now and thinking that you are in a similar place in your life. You may be so overweight that you feel hopeless, just like the young woman in my story. **There is hope! There is always hope! Even though I believe in you, you have a God in heaven ready right now to pour out His power into you so that you can have the *Courage to Change*.** We all need accountability to accomplish healthy goals. Get connected in your church. Start accountability groups and *Courage to Change* Bible studies because the life you save will not just be your own. There is a little boy, or girl, out there who needs you to be ready!

The second story is set in Grapevine, Texas. My friend and colleague Don and I went to a megachurch that seats 15,000 people. At the time, I was in the middle of going through my own major changes as God was showing me the importance of accountability in health, wealth, and virtually every other area of my life. Once the praise and worship stopped, the pastor came out in an apron. I thought it was a great idea. Rarely do you find a church that preaches on health. But as the sermon went on, I felt uneasy, anxious, and frustrated with the message.

Before I go on, I want to say that I believe the church had good intentions. It was a bold move, but because working with people in the fitness arena was out of the pastor's expertise, he fell short of the mark. The pastor showed a pantry of foods and how much sugar was in many of them. That was great. But never once did he make the connection between God's spiritual principles and the behavior that needs to change as a person learns how to eat better and exercise. Halfway through the service, he brought up a local celebrity who had his own chain of health clubs throughout the Dallas metroplex. One of his clubs was just a few miles down the street from the church. The service became an infomercial for his gym.

This was all fine and dandy, but as I looked around I saw thousands of people sitting there seeing something they see every five minutes on local television. Most of the congregation just sat there like zombies, having no idea that the root of unhealthy lifestyle and behavior lies in violating the very principles of God that were taught there every Sunday. I became so frustrated that I was ready to walk up to the front and make a scene because it was clear that the people just weren't getting it. I probably would have been arrested if I had. So instead I began to pray. "What do I do, what do I do, God? These people aren't getting it." While on the edge of my seat, a thought entered my mind. It was as though I were being told to look back behind me down the aisle to my right. As I did so, I saw the most important person in the whole room, the very reason we are to take care of ourselves and fight whatever oppression that keeps us from choosing healthy behavior. There sat a young boy out in the aisle alone in a wheelchair. His head was to one side propped up on a pillow. Clear tubes ran from a machine of some kind up and into his mouth. Here the pastor was talking about nutrition and exercise with a local celebrity, and all I wanted to do was run to that young boy and ask him for forgiveness for every time I ever whined about being too tired to exercise, or complained about being sore from a workout. I wanted to look into his eyes and promise him I would do my best to take care of myself to honor him, to say I was sorry for anything I ever did that was disrespectful to my body and health. I wanted to hold him and cry with him. He will never dance on two feet with a beautiful girl at his prom. He will never know what it feels like to sink a lay-up or go water skiing. He will probably never experience the sheer exhilaration of making love with his wife. It was he the pastor should have had on that stage. It was he who should have been by the side of the pastor as he talked about accountability, which was not discussed.

Every one of us in that room who had full use of our limbs weren't just accountable to ourselves and to each other. Every one of us was accountable to that young boy. I pictured the entire congregation, one by one, looking into the young boy's eyes and asking forgiveness for all the whining and excuses we had made for not exercising and eating right. So many of us have said things like, "I just don't like to sweat." I've heard it a hundred times when talking to people. Can any of us truthfully look into the eyes of this child and selfishly say, "I just don't like to sweat," when this child would give anything for just one day to break free from his wheelchair and run around, jump, leap, crawl and hop until he collapsed from exhaustion? Tears fill my eyes as I think of my own arrogance over the years in taking for granted the health I have been given. If I could change places with that young boy for a week, I would do it in a heartbeat. It would be my pleasure to give him the gift of experiencing "my health."

My heart hurt for the rest of the service. I knew the pastor was trying to teach on nutrition and exercise, and he did a good job as far as it went, but he never addressed the spiritual root of unhealthy behavior. He never talked about the accountability we all have *for* and *to* our children, especially those who are disabled. I sat there not knowing what to do. I felt I had to do something. I began to pray again, "Lord what do I do? If you ask of me, I will go to the front with that little boy." In my mind I heard the word *patience*…that there would be a time I would tell this story, but the time was not then. The seat next to me to the right was empty, and in the one next to it was a young woman I didn't know. I felt compelled to tell her what I was experiencing. So I turned to her and asked her to look back behind her and to the right. She did and saw the young boy in the wheelchair. She turned back to me, and I said to her, "That young boy is the reason we take care of ourselves, so we can honor him through our accountability *to* him. These people in here aren't getting it!" To my amazement she agreed, and I could hardly believe my ears as she proceeded to tell me what she did for a living—she took care of children just like that little boy in the wheelchair. She was a love note from God validating my concerns. We talked more after the service, and she calmed my anxious mind. I looked for the boy after the service but couldn't find him. I wanted to tell him everything I just wrote about.

We are not just accountable to ourselves, but to our children and to every person unable to use his or her body in a functional way. I did not share this story to cause guilt or shame in anyone. Let us all look into the eyes of someone unable to move and say, "I will take care of myself for the rest of my life. I am sorry for my excuses. Please forgive me." Every breath I take, every drop of sweat I shed, and every step I take will, in some way, honor those who cannot do likewise!

Support

Support is the attitude of accountability! One of the greatest components of your success is the quality of support in your life. So many times I have trained women who, shortly after starting an exercise and nutrition program, quit because her husband or boyfriend not only doesn't support her efforts, but worse, sabotages them by his own insecurity and controlling behavior. The woman often hides receipts, my book, and even her gym membership to avoid being cut down by the man in her life. Many women call for help regarding their health, but never follow through after talking it over with husbands who don't support them. So I never hear from them again. Often men feel threatened by their wives' or girlfriends' getting stronger and gaining a sense of self-sufficiency and individuality. The woman loses weight and remains strong for a while, but inevitably quits to keep the peace and avoid conflict. This is an atrocity! Why is it that so many of us, out of our own fear of positive change, do our best to pull others down? Why is it that our greatest fear is not failure, but our own personal greatness? Where is the leadership from the men in this country to support and encourage our wives and children to be their very best, to do what they need to do to break free from unhealthy behaviors and lifestyles?

Sabotage: It is as bad to receive as it is to give. Many of you reading this right now have either (a) been on the receiving end of another person's control and sabotage, or (b) been on the giving end of holding someone else back because of control and fear from your own insecurities. Here is the clincher. Both are equally harmful and equally destructive. Allowing someone to control you and manipulate you into forfeiting your dreams, aspirations, and goals is just as bad as the actions of the one who is doing it. *Don't let anyone stand between you and the dreams God has placed or planted inside of you.* This includes husbands, wives, boyfriends, girlfriends, pastors, parents, siblings, anyone! Sure we are to seek counsel as we reach our aspirations, but through prayer, and more prayer, God will tell you His plans for you. Sometimes they won't make any sense whatsoever to anyone but you, but through your own personal relationship with Christ and His counsel from His Holy Spirit, you can push forward in His will.

If you are one who thinks that maintaining health and fitness is just some vain and time-wasting activity and tells people close to you that they shouldn't waste their time, and that you will not support or pay for it, **stop it! What you are doing is wrong.** God is right there wanting desperately to show you how to be an amazing encourager to others. He also wants to show you the beautiful value of good health and its crucial role in your life and in the life of your family.

I have seen this sabotage over and over in the church as well. It occurs when someone justifies unhealthy lifestyles, and behaviors, by twisting out of context the scriptures that tell us that God looks at the heart, and not the outward or physical appearance, of a man or woman and that physical adornment is wrong. Sure merely *physical* adornment is wrong, but learning to love yourself enough to take action regarding your health and well-being *is* a God thing. It *is in* your heart that God sees you appreciating and loving the gift of life He gave to you. Being a good steward over your life and "your health" is your gift back to him. I have seen pastors weighing 300 pounds preach that health and fitness are vain and a form of idolatry. Pastors are still just people with their own insecurities and fears of reaching new levels of greatness. They need prayer, accountability, and support the same as the rest of us. In my opinion, they need it more because of the position of influence they are in. If anyone needs to be an example of good health, it is the pastor, priest, or minister.

Those of you who have struggled with the support of your loved ones and felt beaten down, know that there is a constructive kind of support. There is help and there is hope. Reach for your greatness and never stop. It may be and probably will be hard, but God created you to be strong and confident through all kinds of trials.

Beware self-sabotage. Make sure that you do not sabotage yourself either. About 50% of my clients over the years who have started an overall program come down with some kind of cold or sickness during the first month of training. Don't expect it, but if it does happen don't let it sabotage your quest for greatness! First, your body is not used to the added physical stress and work. Second, certain behaviors and forces are at work trying to keep you in your old unhealthy way of living. I have seen it over and over again. Many people quit after getting a cold or other sickness. Don't do it! If you think of this as a time of testing and perseverance that you must go through to learn to get and stay healthy, you will push forward regardless of what is thrown at you. Make sure you have the support and accountability you need because old habits (behaviors) are hard to break. You must go through this process to find the root of your behavior (as you will learn in the next section, on knowledge).

We are called to "encourage one another and build each other up" in the Holy Spirit (1 Thessalonians 5:11). We are called to support our fellow believers and the church in many ways. Ministry is a form of support. Tithes and offerings are a form of support. Encouragement is a form of support. A shoulder to cry on is a form of support. Creating abundance means giving and receiving support. Some of us are quick to give support and to encourage others but struggle with accepting support and encouragement ourselves. Many of us are just the opposite. Our ego and pride often get in our way. During your PM reflection time and nightly journaling, part of what God will expose is where you struggle with giving or receiving support. **Support begins with "prayer"—both in giving and receiving!**

Before you can either give or receive support from any person effectively, you must learn to go to the source of all support, to Him who never tires of listening to your dreams, requests, concerns, worries, and thoughts—God himself! He will never make fun of you. He will never laugh at something you take to Him or ask Him in prayer. Many of you may wonder why I do not have an entire section on prayer because of its significance in your life. Well, here's why. If nothing else, this entire book and course is about learning to live your life in a constant state of prayer, at all times, in every situation, every moment of every day. **"Rejoice evermore. Pray without ceasing. In everything give thanks: for this is the will of God in Christ Jesus concerning you"** (1 Thessalonians 5:16–18). Prayer is not just asking God for things or praying for someone else who is in need. It is also being in a constant state of thankfulness and gratitude for the strength and courage He is constantly giving you to conquer every obstacle in your life, including stress of any kind on any level. **"Do not be anxious about anything, but in everything, by prayer and petition, with thanksgiving, present your requests to God. And the peace of God, which transcends all understanding, will guard your hearts and your minds in Christ Jesus"** (Philippians 4:6–7).

But why would God guard your heart and mind (with peace) in Christ Jesus? What is His motive? As you will learn, even prayer must be accompanied by action. A lack of peace paralyzes you and keeps you from taking action. He will guard your heart with peace, show you the way and will answer your prayers, but it is *you* who must walk through the door He opens, whatever that may be and whatever that looks like! The action is yours! *Prayer without action is a selfish attempt to hold God accountable for your success or failure!*

So **"pray without ceasing"** and watch as God becomes the greatest support system in your life. The foundation of a house is what supports the entire structure erected on top of it. But the structure on top of the foundation takes action to build. Every nail, every screw, every board, and every measurement is executed with action by…*you*. Through prayer, Noah was told to build a boat. Noah never ceased in praying, but, who drove every nail and cut every board of the ark—God or Noah? Noah! His prayer was always action. He and God worked together as best friends to accomplish a goal, which inevitably saved his and his family's lives. Set your health atop the foundation of God, the support of God, then take up your hammer and nails and do the work to make your body an "ark," a vessel capable of saving your life and the lives of your friends and family! As they say in AA, "Faith can move mountains…but you better bring a shovel!"

As you think of different ways to both give and receive support, there is one form of support aside from prayer that leads all others, one that sets the stage and has the power to create or destroy! **Your tongue!**

> **"Reckless words pierce like a sword, but the tongue of the wise brings healing."** (Proverbs 12:18)

The scripture here doesn't specify healing of your emotions or your spirit. It is general because it refers to every part of you. Every part of you is interdependent and intricately connected. Every word you say to yourself or others that is not out of love and encouragement is poison to your physical body. It shows up in the form of stress headaches, ulcers, colds, and many other afflictions. What you say comes from somewhere inside you. Jesus once said it is not what goes into a man that makes him unclean, but what comes out of him! What comes out of your mouth begins as a thought, does it not? As you continue working this program in the weeks ahead, you will begin to take captive your thoughts and make them obedient to Christ. As you do this and increase the self-control and love-inspired discipline in your life, you must keep a leash on your tongue.

> **"If anyone considers himself religious and yet does not keep a tight rein on his tongue, he deceives himself and his religion is worthless."** (James 1:26)

Before God got a serious hold on me, whenever I would get upset, angry, or hurt, I cussed like a sailor. I would structure entire sentences with nothing but cuss words and, frankly, I was pretty good at it. I remember a time in college while working at a lumber yard in Kansas when I said every word in the book. I may have even rewritten the book. I had to make a delivery to someone's home with some very expensive paneling. If any of you know the weather in Kansas, you know it gets very hot and very windy. After loading the back of the flatbed truck with the paneling and strapping it down nice and tight, I drove away from the front of the store. Did I mention that the wind was blowing in gusts of about 45 miles per hour that day? Right in the middle of the street, in 107-degree heat, the wind snapped every sheet of that expensive paneling and hurled them down the street end over end. Customers saw it happen. The owner saw it happen. As far as I was concerned, all of God and creation saw it happen. But instead of taking it in stride and dealing with it calmly, as Christ would, I think I would have scared off a terrorist with what came out of my mouth. I didn't realize at the time how such a small thing like my tongue could have such a profound impact on my life. James 3:5–6 shows exactly where I was: **"Likewise the tongue is a small part of the body, but it makes great boasts. Consider what a great forest is set on fire by a small spark. The tongue also is a fire, a world of evil among the parts of the body. It corrupts the whole person, sets the whole course of his life on fire, and is itself set on fire by hell."**

Wow, James's own words are pretty strong, but how true they are. As I longed to know Jesus more intimately and craved the love I felt Him calling me to, I learned to control my tongue and have used it to glorify God. I now want what I say to be beautiful and healing to people, especially those people who hear me when I think I am alone. My thoughts began changing too. Basically, I learned that if I didn't have anything good, and wholesome, and encouraging to say, I was to flat keep my mouth shut!

And when I mess up—and I still do at times, when something bad happens, like when I stub the inside of my pinky toe on one of those hollow, really hard dog bones with the sharp jagged edges from being chewed—and sometimes slip, I simply say I am sorry to God and to whoever heard me and move on with no condemnation or guilt. But it doesn't happen very often anymore because I have trained myself to be self-controlled with what comes out of my mouth. I have learned, as it says in James 3:7–10, that I cannot tame my tongue but can only control it: **"All kinds of animals, birds, reptiles, and creatures of the sea are being tamed and have been tamed by man, but no man can tame the tongue. It is a restless evil, full of deadly poison. With the tongue we praise our Lord and Father, and with it we curse men, who have been**

made in God's likeness. Out of the same mouth come praise and cursing. My brothers, this should not be."

We can control a wild tiger and teach it tricks, but we can never tame it. It is wild and will always be wild. We must always be on our guard when working with a tiger because no matter how good it is at doing tricks, it will always be a wild animal capable of doing harm. Our tongue is no different. As soon as we think our tongue is tame and we get too relaxed with it, we find out that it, just like that tiger, is still a wild thing that can hurt or maul.

Now (most of the time) when my pinky toe kicks the sharp jagged edge of the dog bone and slices the tender skin in-between my toes, I may hop up and down and say or mumble something like "God bless America!!," "Fudge cookies!!," or "Supercalifragilisticexpealidocious!!" I often don't say anything at all. One time I was helping some good friends work in the yard and as I walked in the garage to get something, a huge hornet stung the top of my hand. Man, was it painful. The first thing out of my mouth was the "S" word. It totally slipped out. The kids were shocked because they had never heard me say that before. They teased me about it for quite some time because they knew it wasn't a part of my normal speech. Immediately after it happened, I apologized to them for saying it. Anything remotely profane is damaging to our spirits. Whatever comes out of my mouth greatly affects the people around me, especially children. I want a legacy of healing words of encouragement and life to be left for my family. They learn this behavior and self-control from *me*!

> **"The tongue that brings healing is a tree of life, but a deceitful tongue crushes the spirit."** (Proverbs 15:4)

Let God transform what comes out of your mouth so you can bring healing to your family and friends. Protect your spirit by letting love roll off your lips. As you have learned in the "I Am" section of *Courage to Change*, there are specific ways you should speak to yourself and others. When God speaks, His very voice commands it to be so. God shows us in Genesis how His very voice speaks life into existence!

And **God said**, "Let there be light," **and there was** light. (Genesis 3)

And **God said**, "Let there be an expanse between the waters to separate water from water." **And it was so.** (Genesis 6)

And **God said**, "Let the water under the sky be gathered to one place, and let dry ground appear." **And it was so.** (Genesis 9)

Then **God said**, "Let the land produce vegetation: seed-bearing plants and trees on the land that bear fruit with seed in it, according to their various kinds." **And it was so.** (Genesis 11)

And **God said**, "Let there be lights in the expanse of the sky to separate the day from the night, and let them serve as signs to mark seasons and days and years, and let there be lights in the expanse of the sky to give light on the earth." **And it was so.** (Genesis 14–15)

And **God said**, "Let the water teem with living creatures, and let birds fly above the earth across the expanse of the sky." So God created the great creatures of the sea and every living and moving thing with which the water teems, according to their kinds, and every winged bird according to its kind. **And God saw that it was good. God** blessed them and **said,** "Be fruitful and increase in number and fill the water in the seas, and let the birds increase on the earth." **And it was so.** (Genesis 20–22)

And **God said,** "Let the land produce living creatures according to their kinds: livestock, creatures that move along the ground, and wild animals, each according to its kind." **And it was so.** (Genesis 24)

Then **God said,** "Let us make man in our image, in our likeness, and let them rule over the fish of the sea and the birds of the air, over the livestock, over all the earth, and over all the creatures that move along the ground." **So God created man in his own image, in the image of God he created him; male and female he created them.** (Genesis 26–27)

When God speaks, life and creation happen! As you see in the last scripture above, *you* were created in the image of God and were given the same power through Christ to speak life into existence and follow it with action.

> **"The tongue has the power of life and death, and those who love it will eat its fruit."** (Proverbs 18:21)

I will remind you over and over throughout this book that thoughts, attitudes, speech, and prayer must always be followed by action.

Speak life in and over yourself and all people at all times. Speak confidence and courage into yourself and others at all times and believe with all certainty that God will, and is manifesting it in your life. Everything you see created in the universe was created for *you*, by God, to rule over with love, respect, and stewardship.

Now, for the moment of truth! You must at all times speak truth and health into your physical body. I have never worked with a client with a potty mouth or negative things to say who was truly happy! And, without gaining control over the tongue, rarely did they take back control of their health.

> **"He who guards his mouth and his tongue keeps himself from calamity."** (Proverbs 21:23)

When you speak harmful, degrading, or destructive words into yourself and others, you squelch spirits—yours and theirs. How can you be motivated to take care of yourself if what comes out of your mouth is negative, doubtful, and pessimistic? If you verbally shame yourself, or your family, for doing something wrong instead of speaking forgiveness, life, healing, and encouragement, your **"reckless words pierce like a sword."** Negative, shaming, guilt-inducing speech is worse than simple profanity because it directly projects those words into someone else and pierces his or her spirit. This is called abuse, and it *must* stop!

Here's an exercise to help you actually experience the physiological effects of profanity or abusive speech: Think of the very worst thing you can possibly say. Do that now and sit with it for a moment. You should immediately feel something happen even when you just *think about* the words. This is because they are poison! They stir up negative emotions and squelch your spirit.

Like a dose of liquid poison, they make your body feel bad. Take this exercise a little further: Think of the happiest, most amazing thing in your life, something that puts the biggest smile on your face. Give yourself a moment. I bet you felt something different this time. It was your spirit being fed not squelched. Good, positive thoughts make your body feel good! Now, before that smile fades and while you are still remembering what makes you the happiest, say out loud the negative words or thoughts you thought of earlier. What happened?

Take a moment to think about your experience. It was very difficult to keep your smile, wasn't it? Here's why. Your facial expression is simply the physiological response to what you are thinking and saying! In this case, your thoughts and your words were in direct contradiction with your face! Whether what you thought of was profanity, shaming or ridiculing someone, your body does not want to smile at all while you are saying it. Many of you probably refused to even say it. If what you say is not from love, then your body feels bad and it is difficult to even "fake" a smile. But the more positive words you speak, the easier it is to smile because they make your body feel great! If it is hard to smile while thinking or saying something negative, just imagine how hard it is to exercise. It is nearly impossible because negativity is physically *and* spiritually paralyzing!

How many of you have ever started a diet and exercise program and not had the support of your friends and families? Romans 14:13 states, **"Therefore, let us stop passing judgment on one another. Instead, make up your mind not to put any stumbling block or obstacle in your brother's way."** You are told to **"make up your mind"** (to control yourself) by making sure that everything you do is helpful and nurturing to those in your life. This means paying attention to the needs of yourself and your family members as each of you begins his or her journey toward healthy living. This very much includes your tongue! Those of you who do not have the support you need at home should rely as much as possible on your fellow participants in the *Courage to Change* program and on pastors, church members, and counselors, as well as a qualified spiritually trained personal trainer. We are all here to support and serve you!

To close this section on support, I would like to share with you an experience I had several years back. In the summer of 2000 while at a supercross motorcycle race in Colorado Springs, I witnessed something horrible. I noticed a man sitting down in front of my friends who seemed angry. I leaned over to my buddy and told him I just knew that the man beat his wife or girlfriend. I could tell by his mannerisms and the anger in his eyes. About 30 minutes later, after a few more beers, the man started verbally abusing the woman he was with—all the while two kids were sitting between them. He proceeded to smack her around a bit, which caused me to get a little closer to them. He would take his middle finger and his thumb and flick her ears and head and clench his fists. The whole time she sat quietly with her hands in her lap or held the kids. He smacked her hard enough the last time for me to say enough. I couldn't believe what I was seeing. I was not happy! So I got in between them, placed my hand firmly on his shoulder, looked into his eyes, and sternly told him that he would not touch this woman again and that he would treat her with nothing but respect. I told him I didn't care what problems he thought they had, a woman is not to be touched in any way other than with gentleness and respect. He then proceeded to let me know what he thought of me and offered to take me around back and kick my butt (not the words he used). He bowed out his chest, clenched his fists, and huffed and puffed as I very calmly and confidently informed him, "If that is what it is going to take to keep you from smacking around this woman, let's go! But let me let you in on a little secret. I MIGHT HIT BACK, you coward!" Of course, we didn't go around back. Only a coward smacks a woman around. But you must know that, as a last resort, I would have gone around back to keep him from beating the woman. The cops were called, and I had him arrested. It was up to me because—*surprise, surprise*—she denied the whole thing!

Well, on September 5, 2000 I took a day off work and drove in to Colorado Springs to testify. I figured that if she wasn't ready to stand up for herself and her kids, I would. Many of my friends said it would go nowhere and that he would get off scot-free. One young friend of mine, who had herself been date-raped, also saw no hope. Because of her past experience, she immediately thought it was a waste of my time and that I was a fool to even try. To all of you, I say: *Never, under any circumstances, lose hope!* Let the hope that comes from Christ be your fuel in life. The man received two years of very strict probation and had to report each week to his probation officer. If he so much as breathed on her wrong or even jaywalked, he would go to trial and jail. He was also ordered to attend nine months, or 36 weeks, of spousal abuse counseling and undergo drug and alcohol rehabilitation. Though at the time the woman didn't leave him, a seed had been planted in her that she was worth more than she was getting. She was contacted weekly by counselors, even though she was not ready to talk. I have hope that she, too, began to flourish with life-changing decisions.

Never lose hope! Never lose hope! Never lose hope!

Sometimes in life you may be called to give support to someone who does not want it. The question is, *What will you do?* When you have a chance to make a difference in someone's life, what would you do? In a crowd of strangers, would your belief system and confidence allow you to get involved, or would you stay behind the scenes and do nothing? I truly believe that I saved a life that night. You never know when you just might be the answer to someone's prayers. Believe in yourself and have enough faith in God to make a difference in this world. Stand up for what is right and let people know you care about them by your word and actions that follow. We are all farmers in this world. It is not up to us to make the seeds grow but it *is* up to us to plant them and nourish them! Let us all do our part. If any of you are low in seeds, ask God and He will give you all you will ever need!

And to those of you who think it was foolish of me to exchange words with the abusive man, let us recall the scene when David slew Goliath: **"Goliath looked David over and saw that he was only a boy, ruddy and handsome, and he despised him. He said to David, 'Am I a dog, that you come at me with sticks?' And the Philistine cursed David by his gods. 'Come here,' he said, 'and I'll give your flesh to the birds of the air and the beasts of the field!' David said to the Philistine, 'You come against me with sword and spear and javelin, but I come against you in the name of the LORD Almighty, the God of the armies of Israel, whom you have defied. This day the LORD will hand you over to me, and I'll strike you down and cut off your head. Today I will give the carcasses of the Philistine army to the birds of the air and the beasts of the earth, and the whole world will know that there is a God in Israel'"** (1 Samuel 17:42-46).

Amen! It sounds to me like this is good old-fashioned trash-talking. Goliath tried to steal David's confidence by his words, his posturing, his anger, and his immense size. But what did David do? He basically said, "Are you talking to *me?* Do you know who I am and whom I serve? Not only will I defeat you, but I will cut off your head and feed your dirty carcass to the birds of the air and the beasts of the earth." This means buzzards, vultures, and flesh-eating animals such as lions and tigers and crocodiles. David sounds pretty confident to me. Now please, don't go looking for a fight after reading this. I am not encouraging you to become a brawler, but you must know that there are times in your life when you *must* stand up for yourself and others with a confident boldness. I actually had no intention of fighting that abusive man at the supercross race. All I wanted was for the woman to be safe, and I was willing to take my chances to see that she was. I was ready if he came at me. If standing up for yourself poses a serious risk to yourself or others, then call in the authorities. Dial 911 and let them take care of it! As you speak love and truth into yourself and others, and give and receive support, there is a boldness that you must learn to own. You learn this in detail as you daily practice the "I Am" declaration:

> **The goal of good support is to remind you that God is the great I AM, and through His leadership YOU become the great YOU ARE.**

As you take ownership of God's word by practicing the "I Am" declaration, you will use the same words you own to speak life into your friends and family. You teach them to own the word of God by sharing it with them, or reinforcing what and who God tells them they are. They also learn this by watching you and how you treat yourself.

Leave a Legacy of Love not a Legacy of Lies!

When your children make a mistake, what do you tell them? Do you say, "YOU ARE so stupid, YOU ARE an idiot, YOU ARE pathetic?" Or do you say something like, "YOU ARE so smart and know better than that. What were you thinking?" "Did your actions reflect who YOU ARE, how smart and disciplined YOU ARE?" Which of these responses do you suppose will reinforce a change in behavior? The last two will remind children how God made them smart, intelligent, worthy, and disciplined. Just because their actions may have been wrong doesn't mean you reinforce what happened by telling them how bad they are. This will simply cause them to own a thought and attitude in themselves that they are bad! Their actions or performance will then manifest that bad-behavior mindset you reinforced in them. They will simply perform the way they think and believe THEY ARE! For as Solomon put, **"As a person thinks in his heart, so is he"** (Proverbs 23:7). It is your responsibility to help change their behavior by speaking truth to them in terms of how God made them.

How often have you made a mistake and berated <u>yourself</u> with, "YOU ARE so stupid," or, "YOU ARE such an idiot"? And you wonder why your kids struggle. And where did *you* get it from? Did you grow up hearing, "YOU ARE pathetic, YOU ARE fat, YOU ARE ugly, or YOU ARE worthless?" So many of my clients over the years have struggled with their self-esteem and body image because of how they were spoken to when they were young. They grew up hearing negative words spoken over them and lived their lives reinforcing those negative words through their behaviors, thus keeping the legacy of lies alive in the family. Change your world by first saying, "I AM a winner" and then telling others, "YOU ARE a winner." Every single truth in the "I Am" declaration is there for you to be the **"Great You Are."** Encourage one another and speak only life into the people in your world.

Stand up for your right to be strong and healthy. Do the work, be bold, and support and love one another with love, truth, and kindness.

Knowledge

Knowledge! Knowledge! Knowledge! We are so quick to want knowledge but we don't know the spiritual order of how we receive knowledge from God. People want the answers (knowledge) about how to lose weight and take care of themselves. They want answers (knowledge) about how to heal a marriage in counseling. They want the answers (knowledge) of how to handle their children better or even pull off great business deals. We go to college and fill our brains with knowledge. We read books and get on the Internet to gain knowledge. We watch Dr. Phil or Oprah thinking that if we just listen then one day the knowledge we need and want will be there. All these things can help, but there is more, something much, much deeper.

Knowledge alone is not enough. That is why despite all of the knowledge about health and nutrition and exercise more than 65% of the United States population is obese. That is why despite all the marriage seminars, books and advice columns, the divorce rate in the United States is higher than ever before. With all this knowledge, why are our families torn apart and scattered all over the place? Why do our children need therapy? Why do most people not take the initiative to take action toward a goal once they have the knowledge they need to accomplish it? Could it be that before knowledge can be applied, something else must come first?

There is a beginning to this entire process and it is…humility. Humility is the beginning of knowledge. Proverbs 11:2 states, **"When pride comes, then comes disgrace, but with humility comes wisdom."** Proverbs 24:3–4 beautifully states the rest of the order: **"By wisdom a house is built, and through understanding it is established; through knowledge its rooms are filled with rare and beautiful treasures."**

- **Humility**
  Think of humility as the foundation a house sits on. Humility makes for a teachable spirit and opens the door to wisdom (**"with humility comes wisdom"**).

- **Wisdom**
  Wisdom is then the walls and frame of the house that is built on the foundation (**"By wisdom a house is built"**). *Wisdom is your spirit* that "houses," surrounds, or encapsulates everything inside the house. Wisdom, which comes from your spirit, is the protector of what is in your house. Your spirit is what makes you feel safe as you dive into, expose, and change your behavior.

- **Understanding**
  Understanding is the settling of the house, moving in and claiming the house as your own (**"through understanding it is established"**). *Understanding represents your heart.* Your heart is what takes ownership of the house God has built in you.

- **Knowledge**
  Knowledge is not only what fills the house with rare and beautiful treasures but also what takes out the trash, cleans the house, or removes from the house that which is *not* rare and beautiful "(**through knowledge its rooms are filled with rare and beautiful treasures**"). *Knowledge is the brain* and is always the last thing God teaches us. It is also the most difficult to learn or accept because it is the root of all behavior.

As a person takes his body to physical exhaustion, he is humbled before God, much as he is humbled when fasting. As you humble yourself through exercise, you open your spirit to wisdom, the discernment you need to know that something is wrong or needs work in your life. As you seek His face in this newfound wisdom, He gives you understanding. In this understanding, you are settled or move into the truth about what wisdom has shown you. As you better understand your circumstances and behavior, and the fact that you need to make changes, *then* you are brought to knowledge, the actual root of the behavior you are experiencing. But it all begins with *humility*. Humility is the beginning of knowledge. If we follow the scriptures, we can see that:

> from humility comes wisdom,
> from wisdom comes understanding,
> and from understanding comes knowledge.

Life-change is possible only if your heart is humble because then—and *only then*—are you a vessel open and willing to be taught by the Lord (and people). Exercise creates an atmosphere of humility in your heart, which opens your emotions to a state of healing. Through wisdom and understanding, you get the knowledge you need to change. The problem is that you may not like how painful knowledge can be, so you suppress your emotions and in essence do not allow yourself to be humbled. A person who does not want to look at the hard stuff is basically allowing pride to run his life. Pride, which is the opposite of humility, must be dealt with before any healing can happen. The truth is that unless it begins with humility, then wisdom, and then understanding, we have no idea what to do with knowledge. Remember in Proverbs 11:2, **"When pride comes, then comes disgrace, but with humility comes wisdom."**

Many of my clients over the years have missed out on the final breakthrough during their physical trek to spiritual healing because they miss how spiritual the answer is. All they know is that they want to lose weight, but they don't humble themselves enough to let God expose the cause or root (knowledge) of the emotional pain or circumstances that influenced their poor health choices in the first place. Somewhere, somehow, there was a "spiritual disconnect." In discussing this concept about root behavior with my mother, she was convinced that the root of her unhealthy behavior was onion rings. Well, anyway . . .

Discovering What's Really Eating You...

While studying this concept further, I was reminded of one of my clients in Denver. She first came to me weighing almost 300 pounds. I started training her three times per week, helped her get on track with her cardio and nutrition, and put her on my total program. I could tell right away that there was something deeper that had held her hostage for years, and I waited for the opportune time to approach her with my thoughts. Six to eight weeks into our training, after she had lost her first 20 pounds, she confided in me and shared the root (so she thought) of her obesity. As a child, she had been picked up and driven home from school by a stranger. The stranger hadn't touched her. The very next day the same man had approached her sister after school and had kidnapped, raped, and murdered her. My client took on the trauma inside of her and made herself obese and as unattractive as possible so that nothing like that would ever happen to her. The enemy stole her identity and right of being and feeling beautiful with a lean and healthy body. She would often cry during our sessions, as many of my clients do, when allowing the root of their insecurity to surface. I always handle it with gentle encouragement.

Once this woman reached the 60–70 pound mark of weight loss, I knew it was time to have another talk with her. I shared with her the story about the onion. Many of us have heard the story about the onion, but this time it really hit home. I shared that as long as the skin of the onion is still on, it doesn't sting our eyes, but as we peel away the layers, it exposes the essence of the onion, the nourishing fruit which also happens to sting our eyes. Her body fat was no different from the onion. As she shed those excess pounds, she was simultaneously exposing the "true" root of her obesity, *"the fear of attractiveness,"* as it related to the violation and death of her sister. "Guilt" that she lived and her sister died was also a factor and part of the actual root, but for her, fear of being attractive to and desired by men was the driving force. I told her that as she lost weight, she would begin to feel more attractive and that it would drum up suppressed emotions from her past, emotions that had been physically hidden beneath more than 200 pounds of unnecessary body fat. Like the onion, the closer she came to the essence of her reason for being obese, the more her "eyes" would sting as she faced the trauma of her past. I shared with her that as men began finding her attractive again, she would undoubtedly experience fear and, if she didn't watch out, she could sabotage herself by backsliding into her obese lifestyle to avoid the attention of men.

So we went about our training for another month or so. She had lost a total of about 80 pounds when one day as we were training, she said, "It happened!" I said, *"What* happened?" Earlier that day she had been at the grocery store, and for the first time in decades she noticed a man (other than her husband) flirting with her. She said that she had in fact experienced fear that took her back to the reason she had become so obese. But in that moment she recalled my prediction that it would eventually happen. She remembered my words of encouragement—affirming that she deserved to feel beautiful, sexy, attractive, and confident in herself and that it was time she stopped giving her power away and being controlled by fear over what had happened so long ago. She remembered those words and began owning them for herself. She came to our session glowing from head to toe!

She had not only humbled herself by asking me for help as her trainer, but the actual weekly physical exercise humbled her during every session which allowed her to address the pain of what caused her insecurity. The act of exercise created an atmosphere of humility in her heart which opened her emotions to a state of healing. Her actions and inner work also began to honor God and herself because **"humility comes before honor"** (Proverbs 15:33).

What Humility is Not

Many Christians confuse humility with timidity and passivity. There is a huge difference between the two. Ask yourself where you are, and whether your humility is masked by timidity! Makes you think, doesn't it? Spend some time answering that question. Through true humility, this woman also found wisdom. She became wise and discerning about her behavior and how it needed to change. Through that wisdom she was brought understanding. She began to understand more of why she had made the choices she had and why she had struggled for so long with her weight and body image. It was in her understanding that she became settled as she owned the truth about who she was and what she deserved. As she learned why and continued to take action toward fulfilling her goal, she felt safe as she was given knowledge of the root of why she struggled.

The root was not the actual event—that a man who had picked her up the day before had then murdered her sister. The actual event wasn't the cause. The cause was **fear!** She was so afraid of being attractive and desirable to a man that she had manifested that fear in the form of obesity and spent more than 20 years in bondage to that fear. In essence she gave fear (and some guilt) permission to rule her life and control her. When she gained that knowledge, she was able to clean house or take out the trash (fear of attractiveness) and fill her house with rare and beautiful treasures (confidence, security, beauty, and a worthiness to be physically attractive).

She lost over 100 pounds with me and slowly began taking back the authority that had been stolen from her life. She climbed mountains in Alaska and began to think of herself as sexy and attractive and as a beautiful love offering to her husband. I shared with her the healing power of Jesus and watched her grow daily. I am so blessed to have been a part of her story, her victory!

Your own story may be similar or completely different. The downfall of your unhealthy lifestyle may be from a job layoff, a divorce, unhealthy relationship, unhealthy or unbalanced priorities, the death of a loved one, job stress, or good old-fashioned laziness, which of course has a root of its own. God will eventually show you the root of your laziness, too, but only through humility. After all, laziness is a form of pride and is a selfish "act" of doing nothing. But remember, no knowledge you acquire will do you any good unless you first humble yourself, because without humility you will not allow yourself to change or heal.

Everything you learn about yourself is the result of your increased skill at asking God the right questions at the right times, listening carefully to His answers and putting your godly wisdom, understanding, and knowledge to work. As you reflect, let Him instruct you where to cut immature commitments, low priorities, and anchors that drain you of time and energy. Using the **ASK principle** will keep you in daily fellowship with God.

> **"Grace and peace be yours in abundance through the knowledge of God and of Jesus our Lord."** (2 Peter 1:2)

For Reflection:

In your own words, what is the difference between legalism and accountability?

_____

Describe a time when you have experienced being each of the following and how it made you feel:

Judged:

_____

Judgmental:

_____

Supported:

_____

Humble:

_____

Prideful:

_____

_____

What is the "reason" behind the unhealthy exercise and eating behaviors in your past?

_____

Forgiveness

"Bear with each other and forgive whatever grievances you may have with one another. Forgive as the Lord forgave you. And over all these virtues put on love, which binds them all together in perfect unity."
(Colossians 3:13–14)

Unless commitment and forgiveness run hand in hand in your life, past failures will sabotage your future goals. If you bring your past failures into the present and future, you will create the same pattern of failure every time. You must go to the root and destroy it by burying it once and for all. Other than a reminder of where God has brought you from, those *past failures have no place in your life anymore.* So say bye-bye!

Beginning and ending each day with forgiveness and living each moment with a forgiving heart is absolutely fundamental for both your spiritual and your physical growth processes. All of our hearts yearn for the mercy and forgiveness that can come only from a relationship with Jesus Christ.

The ASK principle will help expose where unforgiveness has crept in. So many of my clients over the years have found that one of the greatest reasons they lost their will to take care of themselves was that they were harboring unforgiveness in the form of resentment, blame, and vengefulness over a past circumstance. They found it to be poison, as though an IV of hatred were stuck in their arm. And once they let it all go with a forgiving heart, the heaviness was lifted. And then, miraculously, they found the will to take the steps necessary to better their health. They learned how to set and keep boundaries against those who could possibly hurt them, but with a compassionate and forgiving heart. As we will learn later, unforgiveness, fear, resentment, blame, and hatred are all paralyzing to your spirit. They keep you from taking action because how can you take action when you are paralyzed? Does this sound familiar?

Not a day goes by that we aren't hurt or offended by someone's words or actions. That is why in the *Life Application Journal* and *Captain's Log,* I provide a convenient place for you to list the people you need to seek forgiveness from and those whom you need to forgive. In some cases, where it is appropriate, you should even contact those individuals and ask for forgiveness with love. Doing this on a daily basis will help you let go of the past and not only live in the present but embrace it with joy!

Treating the *symptoms* of poor health is not enough. We must deal with the *causes* or no permanent changes can occur. When you think back to the original point of your health decline, what were the circumstances in your life? Perhaps you were neglected by a parent or spouse. Maybe you were verbally or physically abused. I have had clients lose control of their health after being raped, molested, neglected, and abandoned. These things are all violations of your body and spirit, and without attention to them, it is likely that they will continually manifest themselves in the form of low self-esteem and poor physical health. You need to understand that healing spiritually is absolutely essential for becoming physically healthy *and healing spiritually means that you must embrace the significance of forgivingness.*

An unforgiving heart means that your focus is on circumstances rather than on Jesus Christ. When you take your eyes off of Christ, you lose your courage, enthusiasm, motivation, desire, and inspiration. The only way you can move forward in your life is to forgive others for their part in your circumstances. Forgiveness frees you from what happened so that it can't hurt you anymore!

And what about you? Isn't it time you forgave yourself? Wiping clean your past also means forgiving yourself. If you ask God to forgive you, but then do not forgive yourself or others, you will not be forgiven. Look into your heart and forgive yourself for your unhealthy past. It is impossible to build up yourself or the body of Christ if you are wallowing in self-guilt and unworthiness. Take God at His word—you are forgiven—and apply this wonderful truth to your life. You are innocent!

"Forget the former things; do not dwell on the past." (Isaiah 43:18)

For Reflection:

Name three people you need to forgive?

_____

_____

Describe how it feels to hold onto unforgiveness. What effects does it have on your body, mind, and spirit?

_____

_____

What do you need to forgive yourself for? How will you do it? What will you do this week to see that it happens?

_____

_____

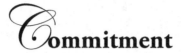ommitment

"A promise or vow fulfilled through covenant"

Now that you are thoroughly excited… Now that you know who you are and where you are going… Now that you have forgiven yourself and others and know just how much God loves you… It is time to make a commitment. Before you begin the section on goal-setting, you must first address the concept of commitment. What good does it do for you to learn about good nutrition, exercise, and setting goals, if you do not understand why you have broken your commitments in the past and why you are making new ones? You may also wonder why we didn't start week 1 with "making a commitment." Good question. I am glad you asked. How can you possibly make a new commitment if you haven't first learned how to conquer the self-defeating thoughts that go through your mind every day? Before making a commitment, you must take back control of your thoughts and attitudes. Now that you have done this and will continually get better at this via the TAP principle and the "I Am" declaration, you are ready to make a commitment.

It is impossible to accomplish goals without commitment. You can think of a commitment as a vow you make to others, to yourself, and to God. Psalm 116:14 clearly says, **"I will fulfill my vows to the Lord in the presence of all his people."** How many times have you broken your vow to take care of yourself? How committed are you right now, and what makes this time any different than all the others? Let's find out. Let's "break" commitment down into the formula shown below. You fill in the blanks to make it represent what you think is the right combination to equal 100%:

(_____)% **Intention** + (_____)% + **Mechanism** (tool) + (_____)% **Results** = 100%.

How important are the three variables given in the formula above? You must *want* to do something, which is your **intention.** The **mechanism,** or *how* you do it, is important. And the **results** you are striving for are also important. Think of each one in terms of its importance and fill in the blank beside each one with a value. Be real with yourself and think as you do this. When you add all three, they should equal 100%. **Don't read on until you have finished the exercise!**

The answer is: **100% Intention, 0% Mechanism, 0% results.** You see, if you truly intend to do something, the right mechanism will appear. As we said earlier in this book, there are many different exercise programs that work great—but only if you intend and commit to work them.

This exercise teaches us that we must put all of our emphasis on our *intention,* rather than on our mechanism or the results. Where have you been spending your time? When I did this exercise, I put 75% in mechanism, 10% in results and 15% in intention. Though I write programs, "how to" books and journals for people, in my own personal life I had trouble finishing things. Because my emphasis was on the mechanism, I would quit or put off something I found wasn't working, or that I had lost interest in. This exercise showed me why. I finish things now because my intention toward a committed goal is 100%.

Jesus: A Man of Absolute Intention

Let's look at the single greatest example of a man's intention to accomplish His goal. Was Jesus' intention 80, 90, or even 99% to die on a cross for our sins? No. If His intention were anything but 100%, He would have stopped because of how hard His goal was. He would have quit, and you and I would not be saved through His love and grace acted out by His shed blood. We are saved because of His 100% conviction or intention to save us. The result is that He died on the cross and came back to us on the third day.

So how do you measure your true intention of something? By the end result you get! If your intention is 100%, the mechanism will appear and the results will follow. You will find a way. Thomas Edison failed thousands of times before inventing the light bulb. If he were here, he would tell us that he simply exposed thousands of ways of how the light bulb *didn't* work. And the mathematical probability is that the more times something doesn't work, the closer one comes to figuring it out. The mechanism or method will always appear. We can measure Edison's intention to invent the light bulb by the end result—he invented the light bulb!

As you embark on this wonderful journey of self-discovery and life-change, frequently measure your intentions by the results that follow. If you do not get the results you want, then ask yourself and God some questions:

- Why are my results not following my intention?
- Is my intention in God's will?
- Is my intention or level of commitment 100%?
- If not, why?
- If yes, have I found the right mechanism? What do I need to change or do differently?
- Do I have limiting beliefs holding me back? (If yes, identify the belief and change it, as previously described in the "I Am" section.)

Commitment is about Covenant, not Emotion

Most of us base commitment on emotion. Wrong! True commitment is not based on emotion, but on **covenant.** Jesus' goal of dying on the cross was based on the covenant He had with His Father in heaven, not on emotion, so He followed through despite how hard it was. You should commit to taking care of yourself by making a covenant between you and God to honor Him with your body regardless of how you feel. As you do this, He will increase your desire and love for what you do because you are doing it for Him.

Think of it like this. Say you take off 50 pounds and keep it off for two years, then gain it back. Was or is your intention 100%? No! If it were, the weight would stay off indefinitely by the mechanism that proved effective for your previous results. You must constantly reaffirm your previous intentions even though you set new ones and have gotten the results you desire. **A true intention of a commitment will not only get you there but will keep you there indefinitely because it is based on a covenant.**

Right now I want you to try your very best to write your name "fast" three times: Really Fast!

1. _____

2. _____

3. _____

Did you "try" it or did you "do" it? Are you going to *try* to exercise and lose weight, or *are* you exercising and losing weight? Are you going to *try* to quit smoking, or *are* you now a nonsmoker? Are you going to *try* to be a better husband/father, or *are* you now a better husband/father?

So many times we use the word "try" as a cop-out to avoid responsibility and break commitments. How many times have you used this term, "Well, I tried"? Of course you tried, and that is why you didn't reach your goal. You didn't DO IT, you TRIED TO DO IT. What happens if someone you do not particularly want to spend time with invites you over to his home for a party? The common response if you don't want to go is, "I'll try to make it" rather than "I probably won't make it," or "No, thanks, I will not be coming." This happens all the time in business. An employer asks for something to get done and the response is, "I'll try to get it done on time." Though the person may very well get it done, he has given himself an out by saying that he will "try." Trying is so often a method for avoiding responsibility and breaking commitments.

Ask yourself how often you use this phrase. How often do you avoid responsibility by giving yourself an out? Learn to be proactive with your decisions and commitments. As Jesus told us in Matthew 5:37, **"Let your yes be yes and your no, no,"** and take responsibility for your commitments and the actions that follow.

While describing the difference between commitment and covenant to Ashley, a client and volunteer firefighter, I was compelled to use the analogy of a fire hose. A commitment without a covenant with God is like a fire hose that is not being held or supported when the water is turned on. The pressure of the water causes the hose to twist and flail violently about and makes it impossible to hit the target and bring about the desired goal—putting out the fire. The pressure of the water that makes the hose fly all over the place represents the pressure of life we experience as we make commitments. Without a covenant with God, there is nothing to hold the hose down (your commitments) so it can put out the fire (your goals). It is actually quite dangerous. In this example, the fire represents something bad, but your goals aren't just about putting out fires. You have beautiful dreams and aspirations that God himself has planted in you. One of them is to be strong and healthy inside and out. He wants to be a part of these dreams and to help make them a reality in your life. By yourself, your commitments are like the flailing hose that flies all over the place and misses its mark. Constrained by a covenant with God, however, lets Him take hold of the hose and aim it so that it hits the mark.

Commitments are parallel (or horizontal), meaning that they go from person to person or even to self, but a covenant with God is vertical. It is the only thing strong enough to make sure a commitment reaches its target.

I made a horizontal commitment to my beautiful wife, Silesia, the day we were married, but that commitment is fulfilled through a vertical covenant with God. My love and commitment to Silesia is based not on emotion or how I feel from day to day, but on a covenant relationship with God. Because of this, I get to see Silesia through Christ's eyes. This means I see her with the eyes of forgiveness, grace, love, and mercy, the same way Silesia sees me. We both mess up from time to time, but our love, anchored by our covenant with God, is steadfast. Though we have made a covenant with God regarding our marriage, we also have one regarding our health. This covenant, too, is based not on emotion or how we feel from day to day. It is based on covenant. Come on now, do you really think that every single workout is the greatest joy of our day? Do you really think that saying no to our favorite extra-loaded crispy-crust supreme pizza with real bacon and pineapple is easy? Guess again! There are days when our workouts and nutrition are based purely on our covenant with God. The discipline (discussed in more detail in week 4) we have for taking care of ourselves is about honoring God and being good stewards over His most basic and beautiful gift to us—*our lives*.

So now we are at the moment of truth. Now that you have read about commitment, are you ready to make one, to God? If you are, on the following page sign, **The *"Courage to Change"* Personal Health Commitment/Covenant** and expect to be held accountable to it.

The "Courage to Change" Personal Health Commitment/Covenant

I hereby commit, or re-commit, my life to God through His son Jesus Christ and in so doing understand that this means taking care of my body and overall health every day with good nutrition and exercise. I understand that though perfection is not possible with any commitment, through the grace of God and this covenant with Him I will do my very best to fulfill this *lifelong* commitment I have just made.

_____

Signed

Congratulations!

Now that you have made a covenant between yourself and God to take care of yourself, it is time to set goals. Though your goals may change and forever evolve, your covenant with God to take care of your health enables you to fulfill your commitments. Forget about the drudgery! Have fun with your health and setting, reaching, and surpassing your goals and dreams.

If you are embarrassed about your measurements, as you begin setting your goals remember this: You are no longer living in the past with guilt, condemnation, and resentment. You are a beautiful child of God. You are living in the *now*, the present, with confidence, self-control, and a renewed Christ-like attitude. It's about the covenant—not about your feelings, so keep your emotions out of the measurements and take each day, each moment, one by one and take care of yourself. God is so proud of you for taking these steps! Press on toward the goal of good health and honor God with your body.

SETTING, REACHING and SURPASSING
YOUR GOALS and DREAMS

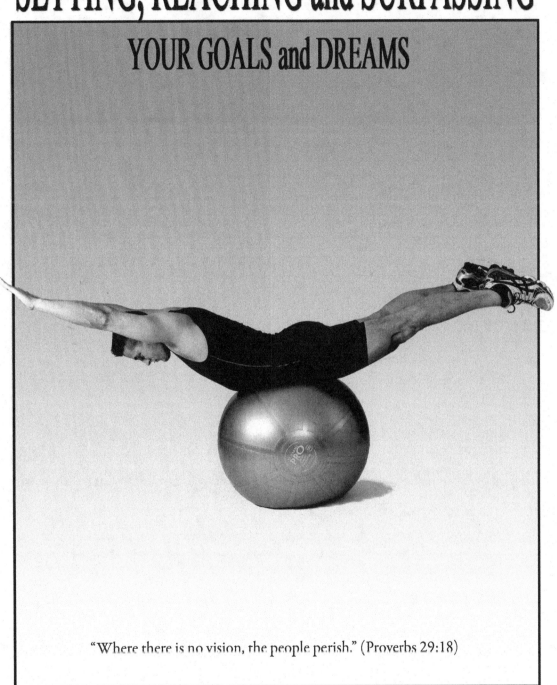

"Where there is no vision, the people perish." (Proverbs 29:18)

WEEK THREE

oals

"I press on toward the goal to win the prize of the upward call of God in Christ Jesus." (Philippians 3:14)

Now it is time to set, reach, and surpass your goals and dreams. Here we go! Jesus not only had courage but a goal. Think of the courage Jesus had as He fulfilled His goal. His goal was to stand in your place and die on a cross for your sins. Like Jesus, you must also have goals. Goals give you aim and a sense of direction. Anytime you are setting goals of any kind, you need to take certain steps to ensure their success. The following five steps should always be part of your goal planning.

I CAN, I WILL, I AM, I DID, WHAT'S NEXT?

Step 1: I CAN = "I can do all things through Christ which strengthens me" *(Philippians 4:13)*. "I can" is claiming a Christ-like confidence and ability toward a committed goal.

Step 2: I WILL = "I will fulfill my vows to the Lord in the presence of His people" (Psalms 116:14). "I will" is setting the commitment or stating a promise and/or signing your name (your word) on a committed goal. Remember your covenant!

Step 3: I AM = "I am the LORD, the God of your father Abraham and the God of Isaac" *(Genesis 28:13)*. God's very voice commands action. (Refer back to the "I Am" section) "I am" is ownership of who you are and is the action that fulfills what the I will promised.

Step 4: I DID = "Do not think that I have come to abolish the Law or the Prophets; I have not come to abolish them but to fulfill them" (Matthew 5:17). **"What God promised our fathers, he has fulfilled for us, their children, by raising up Jesus"** (Acts 13:32–33). Jesus states His intentions of fulfilling the law in Matthew 5:17. His statement is the I WILL, and His life and death is the I AM, and Luke's account of Jesus' resurrection in Acts 13:32–33 is the I DID, or fulfillment of His committed goal of saving you and me. In essence the I DID states the fulfillment of a short- or long-term committed goal or the daily fulfillment of a lifelong committed goal.

For example: Staying loving, gentle, and faithful to your wife or husband is a lifelong commitment that is measured daily. Honoring God with your body through a daily routine is also a lifelong commitment measured daily. Others are goals such as staying sexually pure until marriage, graduating from high school or college, or simply finishing a race you entered. In all of these cases, you must go through all five of these steps, whether the goal is completely fulfilled or not.

Once in a while a goal is not reached at all or at the designated time. In these cases, refer back to the "I Am" section on intention. You and God will find the answer together.

Step 5: WHAT'S NEXT?
"What's next" repeats the previous four steps of reaching a committed goal. What's next means that you are constantly seeking new and exciting ways of challenging yourself to reach the highest degree of excellence in your life. It makes you ask questions such as, "How can I love my wife more effectively tomorrow?" You set a short-term goal to daily fulfill a lifelong commitment to your wife. Now that I have graduated from college, I CAN and WILL find the right job for me. What type of cardiovascular exercise do I want to do tomorrow, different from what I DID today? WHAT'S NEXT takes you right back to:

"I CAN, I WILL, I AM, I DID, WHAT'S NEXT?"

"I CAN, I WILL, I AM, I DID, WHAT'S NEXT?"

"I CAN, I WILL, I AM, I DID, WHAT'S NEXT?"

"I CAN, I WILL, I AM, I DID, WHAT'S NEXT?"

"I CAN, I WILL, I AM, I DID, WHAT'S NEXT?"

"I CAN, I WILL, I AM, I DID, WHAT'S NEXT?"

Let's use the example of weight loss and being healthy as a committed goal. You need to apply this principle to any goal you ever commit to.

I can exercise and eat good nutritious food and be healthy daily and for the rest of my life. **States Christ-like confidence and ability!**

I will exercise and eat good, nutritious food and be healthy daily for the rest of my life. **Sets the commitment or states the promise or vow to fulfill a committed goal.**

I am exercising and eating good, nutritious food and I am being healthy today! It is the action every moment required to fulfill the short-term and long-term committed goal.

I did exercise and eat right today and fulfilled my daily commitment of my lifelong covenant with God to take care of myself. **Either you did, or you didn't!**

What's Next? Maybe your short-term goal is to be able to do 20 pushups without resting, to hire a personal trainer to coach and educate you, and/or to lose 2½ pounds of fat each week. Maybe it is to lower your cholesterol, get off your diabetes medication, or a combination of many others. These short-term goals, whether they are always reached perfectly or always on time, must be part of your long-term goals and lifelong commitment to and covenant with God to take care of yourself. Otherwise, once you reach your short-term goals, you will quit. Short-term goals are simply the building blocks of a long-term goal.

Keep these five principles inside of you. Live by them and remember the scriptures that empower each one. The reason this chapter is so short is because once you have studied all five steps of goal setting, you will need plenty of time to answer and fill out the material in the *Life Application Journal.* Your *Life Application Journal* will address goal setting in detail and will give you an opportunity to get very clear about the goals in your life and how and when you plan to reach them. Go and get the abundance God has in store for you. He will lead you, and through goal setting, He will fulfill His promise to prosper you!

Though a space is provided each week in your journal for recording weekly weight loss, I have provided a chart that goes into a little more detail on measurements. You and/or your trainer can be more specific on your measurements.

Measurements	Start	Wk 1	Wk 2	Wk 3	Wk 4	Wk 5	Wk 6	Wk 7
Date								
Body weight								
Shoulder								
Chest								
Waist								
Hips								
Thighs								
Calves								
Upper arm								
Forearm								
Percent Body Fat								
Resting Heart Rate								
Cholesterol								
Blood Pressure								

Measurements	Start	Wk 8	Wk 9	Wk 10	Wk 11	Wk 12
Date						
Body weight						
Shoulder						
Chest						
Waist						
Hips						
Thighs						
Calves						
Upper arm						
Forearm						
Percent Body Fat						
Resting Heart Rate						
Cholesterol						
Blood Pressure						

LIVING as a DISCIPLE of JESUS CHRIST

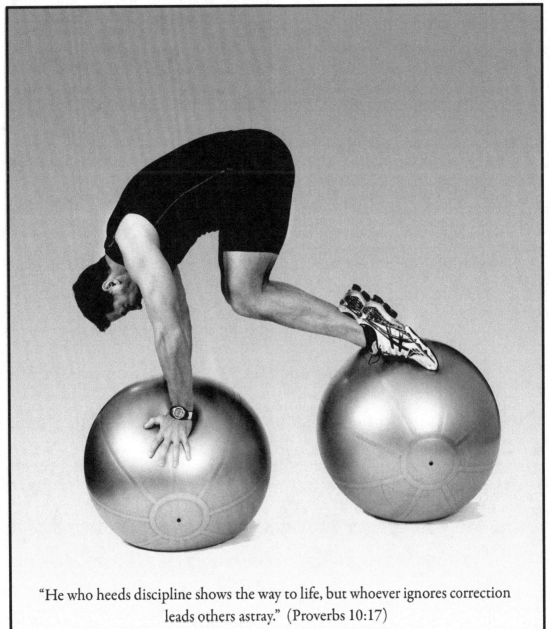

"He who heeds discipline shows the way to life, but whoever ignores correction leads others astray." (Proverbs 10:17)

"For these commands are a lamp, this teaching is a light, and the corrections of discipline are the way to life..." (Proverbs 6:23)

WEEK FOUR

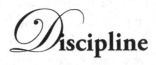iscipline

"Training expected to produce a specific character or pattern of behavior, especially training that produces spiritual, mental, and physical improvement"

Before we dive into the realm of discipline, I want all of you to know that my and Silesia's discipline toward exercise and nutrition doesn't always come easy. Just because we love health and fitness doesn't mean we don't have the same urges, temptations, and crazy schedules that make it difficult to get everything in. While putting the finishing touches on *Courage to Change*, I experienced drastic lifestyle changes. In the prologue, remember those three years of solitude I spent with Christ, during which He changed me. Well, when He felt I was ready and finally opened the door for me, He actually blew the door completely off the hinges. I got married!

Over the course of the engagement and wedding, my lifestyle and time commitments were maxed beyond anything I had ever experienced. I went from a single man living in a one-bedroom apartment to being married with two beautiful children. In a five-month period, I moved from Dallas to a beautiful home in north Houston, planned a wedding and honeymoon with all the trimmings, moved Silesia and the kids once we were married, started a new business, and worked on *Courage to Change*. Did I mention the house needed a lot of work? It needed a new roof, two new air conditioners, two new heaters, and all new toilets. Through all of this, we still had basketball games, school plays to attend, homework, and church activities. I also scheduled as much special time with the most important person in my life aside from God, my bride Silesia. Many of my old clients are laughing right now to learn that I got a huge dose of some of what they were going through. Yes, I have learned the hard way that with children come more snack foods, pizza, and chips. Though we encourage the whole family to eat healthy, and we usually do, we aren't so strict that we don't splurge now and again. But it affected me more because I wasn't used to having fattening or junk foods around the house. Before then, whenever I wanted to splurge, I went out and bought what I wanted, and when I was finished the only food left in the apartment was healthy. Reality check for Brian! Having indulgent foods around all the time has definitely tested my discipline and commitment levels.

During those months of intense lifestyle changes and planning, I gained about 15 pounds. But as I dug a little deeper and allowed God to help me avoid and say no to those amazing orange ice-cream pushups, I found my discipline and balance again, and the extra 15 pounds are now burned away. Let's not even talk about all the butter-cream, raspberry cream cheese wedding cake we took home and put in our freezer. Talk about needing the power and discipline of God! *Oh my!*

The Order of Commitments—To God First, then to...

Part of what my discipline did was keep me in alignment with the Tree of Life, which we will cover later. I couldn't just lose myself in my new family and forget about my health. Has that ever happened to you? I had to stay in alignment and I went through a transitional period where God gave me what I needed to get there. Even with my new family and responsibilities, my health/self had to come first—after God of course. Remember, the self I speak of here is not the selfish or vain kind of self, but the kind needed to fulfill the second greatest commandment, "loving my neighbor **AS MYSELF**." Then came my beautiful wife Silesia, and then our children Shelby and Matthew. How often do kids come before our spouses? This should not happen because it upsets the entire structure of the household and family! My wife Silesia is first and then the children. Then comes work and then additional ministry.

But how often do we—especially we men—put our work and ministry before our children? Our children Shelby and Matthew need a father to step up and take an active interest in their lives. They need to know how important they are by how I make them a priority above and beyond my work. My family is my greatest ministry. It was through my discipline toward honoring God that I kept on track and in alignment. It was hard through that transition period to learn how to juggle it all, but God showed me and gave me the energy. **Remember what the word motivation means? God's energy! See how it all works together?**

Discipline is not a Four-Letter Word

To many people, *discipline* is a nasty word. So many people think of discipline as a military tactic whereby a humorless drill sergeant beats into someone what they need to do by demoralizing them and breaking their spirit. On the contrary, discipline is about love. Why do you discipline your children when they run out in the street without looking? Why do you discipline your children when you know they are doing something that can harm them? You do it because you love them! But this form of discipline results from doing something wrong. Is there another form of discipline? Yes.

Discipline comes from the word *discipleship*. All of us who have welcomed Him into our hearts and want to please Him because we love Him are disciples of Christ. True discipline actually keeps us from doing wrong and keeps us from ever needing the other form of discipline (i.e., when we mess up). **True discipline is not a form of punishment but an act of obedience to strengthen us and keep us out of harm's way.** So, what is the result of disciplining ourselves to exercise? The result is a strong and healthy body with a confident mind and secure emotions. The discipline required to fulfill the need to exercise indeed keeps us out of harm's way, does it not? In its true sense, discipline is a beautiful thing because it teaches us how to be self-controlled in an uncontrollable, crazy world.

Our society has very little discipline. The Bible states that the act of physical exercise profits little compared with how we spread love, but the discipline required in the process of taking care of ourselves is very much a part of what it means to be "disciples" of Christ and also teaches us self-control. **"For God did not give us a spirit of timidity, but a spirit of power, of love and of self-discipline"** (2 Timothy 1:7). You can't find these qualities outside of yourself. God clearly states in the scripture above that He has already given you these things. Reach inside yourself and pull out the amazing person you have caged up for so long. Break free from the bondage of self-doubt and insecurities. Live and act with power, authority, love, and self-discipline.

Many food and drug addictions begin with a lack of self-control and self-discipline. Self-control is a fruit of the Spirit and one of the most important results of taking care of ourselves physically. You can overcome these and other dangerous behaviors with authority and love, knowing that the blood of Christ has already made you worthy to be strong and healthy in all areas of your life.

A Family Affair

So how do you start exercising this discipline God has given you? One way is by taking a *family* approach to it. How many families nowadays actually sit down and have dinner together? Most kids come home and fend for themselves or grab their plate of "unhealthy" food and go sit in front of the TV or video game system. What happened to our family unit? What happened to leading our family by example and teaching what is really important in life—love and togetherness? One of the greatest tools of our enemy is to separate us from one another. We see this division not only on a corporate level between the different branches or denominations of Christianity, but also in the homes of Christian believers.

We have become so separated as a church body—both in our churches and in our homes. One way to restore the lost unity is by having meals together—breakfast or dinner, if not *both!* As you sit down with your family to eat a healthy dinner, you are disciplining your family to take notice of several things: the importance of eating healthy food, which is loving ourselves and honoring God, and being with the family and building relationships with each other, which again is about love and honoring God.

As far as exercise, when you discipline yourself to go exercise, you are teaching your entire family about the importance of being healthy, energetic, and physically active. **"He who heeds discipline shows the way to life, but whoever ignores correction leads others astray"** (Proverbs 10:17). An important question to ask yourself is what role you are playing in the overall health of your family. Are you contributing to your children's obesity, or, are you teaching them with your own actions how to be healthy and physically mature? Are you foolish in doing whatever you want to your body and permitting your children to do whatever they want as well? **"But fools despise wisdom and discipline"** (Proverbs 1:7). These are pretty strong words, aren't they? But again, they aren't my words. I'm only the messenger! I serve the same holy and loving God as you and read the same Bible. God holds us accountable for our actions because He loves us. I hold my clients accountable because I love them (you). The Bible clearly states, **"He who ignores discipline despises himself, but whoever heeds correction gains understanding"** (Proverbs 15:32). Some Bible translations state that to hate discipline is to hate yourself.

For those of you with no discipline this is a wake-up call to take care of your body and those of the ones you love. How in the world are your children going to learn how to take care of themselves and honor God with their bodies if you, their parents, have no discipline? How will they ever learn the true value of what God has given them if they do whatever they want whenever they want and desecrate God's most basic and precious gift to them, their physical body? As you can see, true discipline is about love, *not* punishment. **"For these commands are a lamp, this teaching is a light, and the corrections of discipline are the way to life"** (Proverbs 6:23). Discipline protects you and your entire family from harm and makes you strong, self-controlled individuals.

"He who ignores discipline comes to poverty and shame, but whoever heeds correction is honored" (Proverbs 13:18). Poverty in this context is referring merely to financial poverty but means also sickness, disease, and physical disarray. Sexual immorality leads to sexually transmitted diseases (STDs). Smoking and using other drugs leads to lung cancer, heart disease, emphysema, and many other sicknesses. Overeating and underexercising leads to obesity, diabetes, heart disease, and osteoporosis. So many of our sicknesses are caused by the lack of discipline in our lives. If you have lost track of taking care of yourself, along with sickness and poor health, you probably also feel somewhat "shameful" and guilty, insecure and timid. These feelings do not come from God, and it is time for you to exercise your authority and begin to **"honor God with your body, making it Holy and pleasing to God. This is your Spiritual act of worship"** (Romans 12:1). After all, **"Do you not know that your body is a temple of the Holy Spirit, who is in you, whom you have received from God? You are not your own; you were bought at a price. Therefore honor God with your body"** (1 Corinthians 6:19-20).

For Reflection:

What are some of the ways you have demonstrated a lack of self-love?

_____

_____

What is the difference between punishment and discipline?

_____

_____

Discipline and Self-Control

Is there a difference between discipline and self-control? The answer is YES! There is a big difference. When you read the fruits of the Spirit in Galatians 5:22-23, you will find self-control but not discipline. Why? I, like many of you, used to view discipline and self-control as the same thing. But the more I study the more I see that they are completely different. Discipline is something you demonstrate out of obedience, a *choice you make* to honor God, your family, friends, and yourself.

Self-control, on the other hand, is not something you give yourself or something you demonstrate by what you have on your own. Read this next sentence carefully: Self-control is something only *God gives you* as you choose Him and walk in obedience. The Bible says that obedience is even better than sacrifice, and as you demonstrate your obedience through your actions of love and kindness toward yourself and others, God will impart self-control to you as the fruit or reward. In essence, when you follow Jesus and show yourself obedient through your own discipline, He takes over. Once He takes over, *your* obedience comes from self-control that only *He* gives. Understanding this difference between discipline and self-control not only shows the love God wants *to give you but also the love he wants to receive from you!* It is a two-sided loving relationship; a love affair takes *two* partners!

So how in the world does this relate to your health? When you begin eating right and exercising to honor God, your families, friends, and yourself, you must demonstrate discipline to be consistent. Do you remember what discipline is? *DISCIPLESHIP!* God wants His children healthy and will ask you to walk in obedience through a disciplined lifestyle. But here is the beauty just waiting for you to grab hold of! As you consistently demonstrate your obedience through your own discipline to take care of yourself, the result is the fruit of self-control. You and God walk together in your health as you give to each other. You give Him your discipline out of love for Him, and He gives you self-control out of His love for you! As a bonus, self-control is much easier than discipline because self-control comes from God, whereas discipline comes from you! He wants you to succeed even more than you do! He is beautiful! Embrace Him.

There are four—and only *four*—areas in your life in which God asks for your discipline and promises to give you the fruit of self-control. These four are discussed in detail throughout this book.

1. Eyes and Tongue—As you discipline your eyes and tongue out of reverence to God, He will give you self-control. Remember the tongue is like the rudder of a ship. The rudder is such a small part of a ship, yet it directs the vessel either to safety or destruction. Think of your eyes as the wind blowing the ship in one direction. Even if the rudder is strong, a hurricane will blow the ship wherever it wants. In essence, undisciplined eyes and tongue will lead to sexual impurity, poverty, obesity, and broken relationships, all relating to the following three disciplines.

2. Sexual purity—Sex is perhaps the greatest physical pleasure known but must be experienced only in the context of its original design—between husband and wife. Making love is the closest and most vulnerable two people will ever be together and is the physical act God looks at that consummates (makes official) the marriage of a man and woman, making them one flesh. It is the single greatest act of God's love shared by a husband and wife. Sexual impurity leads to poverty, poor health, and physical and spiritual brokenness. How, you ask? Ask the person paying child support for three different families how hard it is financially and ask the person with AIDS, syphilis, herpes, or gonorrhea if an active promiscuous sex life has affected his health!

3. Financial—Financial discipline is the only discipline God actually says to put Him to the test on. As you prove your faithfulness to God through your tithe of 10% of your increase He promises to bless you. In addition to the tithe God also tells us to not go into debt. Just because you want something "cool" doesn't mean you can afford it. Lack of financial discipline leads to a great many problems. Marital problems often arise because part of a person's sense of safety is tied to the family's financial security. Debt creates stress and often focuses our attention on material things instead of on God and the relationships with people in our lives. Let's put it in perspective. As you are paying off that Hummer, 60-inch plasma TV, 10,000-square foot house, and 40-foot cabin cruiser...who has the time *or* the money to invest in your health? You'll go into debt to purchase something you don't need, yet you won't buy good nutritious food or fitness training because "it costs too much!" Exercising financial discipline is one of the great ways to put your life priorities in order. Once you have taken care of your health and the health of your family, paid your tithe as well as invested in your kids' college fund, if there is enough left over to buy the Hummer with cash...by all means get the yellow one!

4. Health and fitness—Taking care of yourself is, or should be, the most <u>fundamental</u> discipline. The action required to eat right and exercise is a catalyst that will help develop a disciplined "lifestyle." Eating healthy meals as part of a good nutrition plan is a discipline. Exercising is a discipline. Your ability to "actively" love others is largely dependent on your willingness to take care of yourself. Being undisciplined in your health leads to obesity, diabetes, heart disease, emphysema, hypoglycemia, increased allergies, and a whole slew of other problems. God doesn't want that for His children. Do you want that for yours? Does that sound like living an abundant life? I think not!

Each one is part of the other. They all overlap! Being disciplined in these four areas will do one thing...create abundance in your life—physical and fiscal abundance and relational abundance. It is God's promise to each of us.

For Reflection:

Pinpoint which of the following areas of your life you need to exercise discipline in and pray for self-control in. For each one, list how:

Eyes & tongue:

_____

Sexual purity:

_____

Financial:

_____

Health & fitness:

_____

This week, exercise discipline and pray for self-control. Write your prayer below:

_____

_____

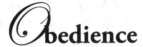bedience

"A love affair with Jesus Christ"

You have learned how to TAP into God by aligning your thoughts, attitudes, and performances with Him and then owning His truth by using the I AM declaration. You have learned how to apply these principles to numerous stressful situations and change your outcome by turning to Christ and His truth. But what is the reason we do all of this? What is the ultimate reason we learn these wonderful principles?

> **The ultimate goal of your *Courage to Change* is obedience, not because you are supposed to obey but because it naturally flows from you unconsciously from your love affair with Jesus Christ.**

While training in Grapevine, Texas, a 38-year-old man who was going to try out as a placekicker for a professional football team called me up for some help getting him into shape. He was also a part-time minister with a true passion for the Lord. In one of our many incredible spiritual conversations during our training, he asked me what I thought obedience was. I answered him with the textbook definition—saying that it consisted of those things we do or the godly principles we follow for ourselves and each other that are biblically or scripturally sound. Obedience is basically following the guidelines as God has set in the Bible. My client looked at me with soft, kind eyes and I could see in his face that he wanted to show me something, something wonderful. He didn't judge my answer as either right or wrong but said that he wanted me to consider it another way. He came up close to me and put his hands up around his eyes as if he were looking through a tunnel and softly said to me, "Obedience is one thing and only one thing: **a love affair with Jesus Christ.**" See, obedience is tunnel vision with Christ as your filter. If you see everything first through Him, then your actions, your thoughts, your attitudes, everything will come into alignment with God.

Jesus' Perfection is Good Enough for God

This was a breakthrough for me. Many of the stories I share in this book are about my overcoming perfectionism—the mistaken belief that my obedience must be perfect for me to be acceptable to God. I used to think I got close to Christ through my actions. *Wrong!* I learned that this was far from the truth—in fact it was a lie inspired by the enemy. To help you understand, extend your arm and hold it out in front of you and picture Jesus in your hand. Let's say the things you do—or your obedience to Him—is your arm, which grows outward to get you to God, which you are holding in your hand. Then bring your hand in as close to your face as possible so that all you can see is your hand, which represents Jesus. Now, you are free to do the things you need to do because they are coming from Jesus. He becomes the filter that everything in your life passes through. The things you do are not what get you *to* Christ—they come *from* Christ. Then *and only then* is your **love affair with Jesus Christ made manifest in your actions.** In your actions you are free, because with Jesus as your filter you receive His grace. He looks at us—those who believe in Him—not with disappointment because of our imperfections but with total acceptance and perfection because of His sacrifice for us. He is proud of us and loves us *not* because of what we do or how we do it—He is proud of us and loves us because we are His children. In *that* love affair we now freely spread His love wherever we can. In *that* love affair we are free to take care of ourselves on *all* levels.

If perfection is your aim, you can go crazy trying to figure out exactly what principles to follow and the right interpretation of scripture in order to be "perfectly" obedient and *earn* God's love. That is why Jesus came—to show how to change the "thou shalt not" to the "thou shalt." He turned the moral codes from negative to positive. Instead of "Thou shalt not murder," Jesus said "Thou shalt love thy neighbor as thyself." Though the "thou shalt not" commandments are still very much a part of our walk, the new covenant under Jesus changes the emphasis from the negative to the positive. He shows us how to live instead of how *not* to live.

So what does this have to do with your health? A lot! Our society places so much importance on physical appearance that most of us actually seek acceptance from others and measure our value by the shape we are in physically. Television commercials, movies, sit-coms, radio shows, magazines, and virtually every form of media plays on the human body and dictates what is acceptable and unacceptable. How many of you reading this right now place your value in your health or in your physical appearance? How many of you base your self-esteem on your willingness or unwillingness to take care of yourself?

You see, taking care of yourself is definitely an act of obedience, but do not make the mistake of thinking that it will get you closer to God. It will not ultimately give you the joy you want in life, and it certainly will not fill all the holes you thought it would. Could this be a reason you cannot seem to stay focused or committed once you have started a health program? No amount of "doing-ness" or obedience in your life can get you closer to God, **"for if righteousness could be gained through the law, Christ died for nothing!"** (Galatians 2:21)

> **"You, my brothers, were called to be free. But do not use your freedom to indulge the sinful nature; rather, serve one another in love. The entire law is summed up in a single command: Love your neighbor as yourself."** (Galatians 5:13–14)

Your intimate personal relationship with Christ **gives birth** to your obedience, which includes your willingness to take care of yourself! You don't get your confidence from the healthy actions you take; you get your healthy actions from your confidence, which comes from God. You don't get your motivation from losing weight; you lose weight based on your motivation, which comes from God! You don't get your enthusiasm from your willingness to exercise; you get your willingness to exercise from your enthusiasm, which comes from God! You don't become brilliant because you read books and study; you read books and study because you are brilliant, which comes from God!

You don't become great because of the great things you do; you do great things because of your greatness, which comes from God!

Four Steps of Obedience

Remember: "You, my brothers (and sisters), were called to be free." But there are processes you must go through as you let Christ change you and teach you how *not* to "use your freedom to indulge the sinful nature, rather, serve one another in love." There are four steps or levels of obedience He takes you through because He loves you. Christ does this as you apply all the principles you have learned and grow in your love affair with Him.

Level 1: Unconscious Disobedience

Unconscious disobedience is when you are unknowingly living outside of the will of God—perhaps because you are not yet aware that you are doing so. This includes thoughts, attitudes, and performances (TAP). Perhaps there is fear, distrust, or even resentment that you have bottled up inside over some past hurt or a stressor that you do not realize is still hurting you. Virtually every lie in the "I Am" section that you unknowingly live in is an example of unconscious disobedience. God clearly states in Hosea 4:6, **"My people are destroyed for lack of knowledge."** A lack of awareness or knowledge steals your joy, kills your will to do anything healthy, and destroys the very relationships God has put in place for you to prosper.

Level 2: Conscious Disobedience

Conscious disobedience happens when you become aware that a behavior in some area of your life is out of the will of God, yet continue in it. You know it is wrong but you continue to do it—perhaps because you do not yet know how to overcome it. Virtually every lie in the "I Am" section that you knowingly live in is an example of conscious disobedience. You become aware of your misbehavior but don't yet know how to overcome it—this is conscious disobedience. This is a natural progression of how God changes us, and it is why we are to have compassion for and love people wherever they are because we do not know where they are in their progression of obedience. Maybe they are truly seeking God's face but have not figured out how to overcome the disobedience they are consciously choosing. Humility is the key to transitioning from one level to the next. In your love affair with Jesus He will show you in what ways your thoughts, attitudes, and performances (TAP) are out of alignment with His will. Remember the order in the knowledge section? It begins with humility! Through humility God will show you where you have unconscious disobedience. But God is not going to hurl you into the lake of fire because of it. He is a loving Father and, through your humility, He will show you how to change so that you can move to the next level in your walk. He gives you wisdom, then understanding, and then knowledge.

Granted, if a person takes 15 years to stop hitting his spouse because he says he is "in the natural progression of conscious disobedience," something is wrong. This fellow needs to be locked up and smacked upside the head, and not necessarily in that order! For the person actively pursuing a love affair with Christ, Level 2 of conscious disobedience won't take very long. God will place in you so much conviction that you will not want to stay there because it is in direct violation of your spirit.

On occasion I have heard people even pull out scripture to justify their conscious disobedience. One popular scripture is Paul's statement in Romans, **"I know that nothing good lives in me, that is, in my sinful nature. For I have the desire to do what is good, but I cannot carry it out. For what I do is not the good I want to do; no, the evil I do not want to do—this I keep on doing. Now if I do what I do not want to do, it is no longer I who do it, but it is sin living in me that does it"** (Romans 7:18–20).

I briefly worked with a man who cited this scripture every time he talked about his struggles with pornography and pot smoking. He constantly chose conscious disobedience as he engaged in those activities and, to justify his struggles, would remind me what Paul said in this passage in Romans. I have seen this verse used to justify a person's unhealthy habits and all kinds of destructive behavior. Sure, Christ takes us through a process in delivering us from addiction and the other trappings of our sinful nature. God is patient with us and will always pursue us. But I do not believe for a second that this is the behavior Paul was talking about in Romans 7. Paul was in an amazing love affair with Christ. Paul always spoke of his "sinful nature" and "struggles with fleshly desires" with great humility. He did not do so concerning his conscious disobedience (i.e., things that he refused to give up). The things he wrestled with in his flesh were such things as momentary flashes of anger, impatience, distrust, and even simply having a negative thought once in a while. I believe that if he accidentally cussed because he smashed his thumb building a tent, he would immediately be under conviction to change his tongue because of his love affair with Christ. He probably did slip once in a while in various ways—he was human after all—and these slips were what he was writing about. He was just an imperfect man doing the best he could to take captive his thoughts and make them obedient to Christ. He was not willfully living a life of sin and shirking responsibility for it by flippantly saying, **"It is no longer I who do it, but it is sin living in me that does it."** His number one priority was to love Christ and to do the best he could to live his life as Christ would. So, please, do not use this scripture to justify unhealthy behavior. Humble yourself enough to accept that what you are doing is wrong and let Christ transform you as you let Him pour out His love into you. But it is *you* who must act on those changes! It is *you* who must have the *Courage to Change*.

Level 3: Conscious Obedience

Conscious obedience is taking your knowledge of negative or disobedient thoughts, attitudes, and performances (TAP) and making a conscious choice to change them. Virtually every lie in the "I Am" section that you consciously change to the positive and live accordingly is an example of conscious obedience. Moving into conscious obedience is difficult because it requires retraining and breaking bad habits and unhealthy behaviors you have been living in. This is where it sometimes hurts. No, this is where it *usually* hurts! You are going from the familiar to the unfamiliar, from known territory to unknown territory, and it takes a lot of humility and perseverance to stay there.

This level is where God prunes you or trims the branches off your tree that don't bear fruit. Remember Charlie Brown's Christmas tree in *Peanuts*? When I first made the choice to consciously choose obedience in every area of my life, the Lord pruned and snipped and nipped and cut until

I was naked with one little branch. *Ouch!* But now I have more fruit than I ever had because of my love affair with Jesus. This is also where He takes the world out of you or refines and purifies you, as it says in Malachi 3:2–3: **"For he will be like a refiner's fire or a launderer's soap. He will sit as a refiner and purifier of silver."** His goal is to free you from anything that is keeping you from His treasures and to purify you and change you into the likeness of Christ! Many of you may remember how the Bible tells us that we must be crucified with Christ: **"Those who belong to Christ Jesus have crucified the sinful nature with its passions and desires"** (Galatians 5:24). This cannot happen with any part of your life *until you consciously choose* a love affair with Christ. And remember: Your obedience doesn't get you closer to Christ. Rather, it is your love affair with Jesus Christ and the freedom He brings that gives birth to your obedience. It is a beautiful thing!

While on this level, He will show you more and more areas that must be changed. Throughout your entire life, He will constantly bring to your awareness thoughts, attitudes, and performances (TAP) you are unconsciously having or doing that are out of His will. He will then take you through the four levels of obedience to get you back on track. It isn't just one big bang and *poof!* You are changed. It is a process that takes time. The onion has many layers, and God peels it away slowly so you don't miss a thing. It is a moment-by-moment, hourly, daily, weekly, lifelong process of consciously choosing a love affair with Jesus Christ!

Level 4: Unconscious Obedience

Virtually every truth in the "I Am" section that you unconsciously live in is an example of unconscious obedience. Your goal is to be transformed so that your every thought, attitude, and performance (TAP) is unconsciously in alignment with God. This is where your obedience becomes habit—it is a part of you, and you don't have to consciously choose it to accomplish it. You are able unconsciously to TAP into God even as the world around you hurls fiery darts at you. Living in this level is true freedom and gives you a peace that transcends all understanding (Philippians 4:7). This is when the once snipped and pruned branches of your tree grow back and become lush and bear fruit. This is what Charlie Brown's Christmas tree looked like *after* it was decorated. This is where you pick your battles because most of them are won without your even realizing it.

Let's say that one day through your humility and love affair with Christ, God shows you that you have not forgiven someone for something he or she did a long time ago and have been carrying that pain and resentment around with you ever since. The unforgiveness you have been unaware of and living in is an example of unconscious disobedience. Until you sincerely and consciously choose to forgive that person with the knowledge you now have, you are choosing unforgiveness, which is conscious disobedience. But as you grow in your love affair with Christ, He will place in you the forgiveness you need to let go of whatever happened. As you choose forgiveness, you move into the level that actually changes you—conscious obedience. Remember, Christ wants to break and even destroy the yoke of unforgiveness in your life because it is poison to your physical body, your mind, your spirit, everything! His goal is to move you into unconscious forgiveness toward the person who hurt you so that you can love that person even though he or she may be your enemy. You can (and sometimes *should*) set boundaries within your relationships with people who have hurt you, but in conscious obedience you will do so with forgiveness and a loving heart.

If someone has done something atrocious, you can still love and forgive him as he goes to prison and serves his sentence! Forgiveness does not mean forgoing justice!

> **Consciously choosing forgiveness frees you from the violation so that it can no longer hurt you!**

Simply replace the word *disobedience* with *unforgiveness* and watch how Christ takes you through the different levels of obedience. It looks like this:

1. **Unconscious unforgiveness**
2. **Conscious unforgiveness**
3. **Conscious forgiveness**
4. **Unconscious forgiveness**

Virtually every lie in the "I Am" section can be applied to the four levels of obedience. Let's take distrust as an example. The very second you learn that you are having a trust issue, you go to the I AM and own the truth of God by saying, "I AM trusting in the Lord." If it is your husband or wife, then you can say, "I AM trusting my husband or wife." In cases where the other person isn't trustworthy, this will require a different kind of trust. The distrust I am speaking of now is one that prevents you from having a trustworthy relationship. My wife Silesia and I are called to trust each other as an act of obedience. We are a part of each other in everything we do. If there is a past hurt keeping us from trusting each other, through humility God will take us through the levels of obedience to heal. Distrust is poison in our relationship, and we don't want anything to keep us from experiencing the fullness of God's love in our marriage. The sequence looks like this in each situation where trust is an issue:

1. **Unconscious distrust**
2. **Conscious distrust**
3. **Conscious trust**
4. **Unconscious trust**

Choosing trust frees you from the past so it can no longer hurt you!

One area of my life that changed most drastically as I grew in my love affair with Christ was my sex life. Through my youth and young adulthood, the world proclaimed that sex before marriage was fine and a natural part of healthy relationships. When I started going to Spirit-filled churches, I learned that premarital sexual activity of any kind was out of the will of God. I couldn't quite grasp it, though, because I felt that sex in a healthy relationship was about love, the very thing the Bible was all about. But to honor what I was learning, I tried many times to refrain from having sex with girlfriends whom I felt I loved at the time—and failed. The reason I failed so miserably was because my obedience was law-based not Christ-based. I didn't know at the time that there was actually more to my faith than just believing strongly in God. Although I saw God working in my life and even loved Him, I didn't understand the intimacy He wanted with me. But I kept feeling Him tapping me on the shoulder, telling me that there was so much more to my faith in Him than just believing in Him. Only after I surrendered to His love through a relationship with Him did He open my eyes to the truth of why premarital sex was wrong. Only through my love affair with Christ was I strong enough and humble enough to be taught the amazing beauty of abstinence, the true beauty of a woman. I didn't wait merely because I was *supposed to*.

God showed me the amazing beauty and fragility of a woman whom I was to honor and respect. I learned to serve my future wife even before we were together by putting God's desires before my own. It was this honor and respect that drew Silesia to me. I had never honored a woman like that before, and Silesia had never been honored by a man like that before. It was not a law commanding me "thou shalt not have premarital sex" that changed me. That legalist attitude without a context of understanding actually caused me to fail many times. Rather, God convicted me of the truth about how to honor and truly love a woman through my love affair with Christ. My obedience came *from* Him, it didn't get me *to* Him! All this to say: **You cannot "be free" to obey any Godly principle without a love affair with Jesus because only He can open your spiritual eyes!**

Once I focused solely on my love affair with Christ, He took me through all four levels of obedience in regard to sexual purity. In only a few months' time, I surrendered having sex until my wedding night, including any and all other forms of sexual intimacy as well. Though my actions changed, the conscious disobedience occurred as I struggled with changing my thoughts and attitudes. My love affair with Jesus in this area was a process, and my eyes sometimes strayed out of habits that needed to be changed. I learned that even my eyes can sexually take me somewhere I shouldn't go if I don't look through the eyes of Christ. Even looking at a woman in an inappropriate way is disrespectful and dishonoring. After six months of consciously choosing to honor God and my future wife in this way, it became an unconscious behavior. I didn't even remotely desire having sex before marriage because of the love and honor God showed me. Granted, I am a man and my body still felt urges, but never did I desire to act on those urges with anyone besides my future wife. I took my thoughts and attitudes captive and made them obedient to Christ. It became unconscious obedience and four-and-a-half years later, I was married to the woman of my dreams, my soul mate Silesia. The sequence went like this:

1. **Unconscious sexual impurity**
2. **Conscious sexual impurity**
3. **Conscious sexual purity**
4. **Unconscious sexual purity**
   (The topic of lovemaking and sexual purity and their importance to your health is discussed in more detail in Week 12 on "Making Love.")

So how else does the vast spectrum of disobedience appear in our relationships? One day after school I helped our 10-year-old, Matthew, get started mowing the lawn. He had mowed the lawn only a few times on his own. After he finished the front yard, he started moaning and groaning about how tired he was and how he just couldn't finish. I kept asking him what was wrong and he kept telling me the same thing—that he was too tired to finish. So we kept bumping heads. This went on for a while and I got frustrated. I thought he was just being stubborn because he did not want to mow the lawn. My voice got stern and even a little sarcastic as I pleaded with him to finish. He didn't have much of the yard left, but he just would not get his body moving to get it done. As I shared the incident with my wife Silesia she just asked me if I had asked why he was so tired. Matthew wouldn't give me an answer. Though Matthew definitely has his moments,

Silesia reminded me that it wasn't in Matthew's character to whine and fuss over something like that. She also gently reminded me that Matthew had been up half the night for various reasons and wasn't quite himself, probably because he was exhausted.

So I took her words and my ego to the Lord. As I humbled myself, I realized that the frustration I was feeling really wasn't because Matthew wasn't finishing the yard the way he normally did. My frustration came from my unconscious disobedience of my own pride and lack of listening to his needs. In truth, it was out of his character to act that way in that situation. So for a few brief moment as I talked to him, I still had a tone in my voice because I didn't want to let go my pride. At this point I had moved from unconscious pride and lack of listening to conscious pride and lack of listening. But as I humbled myself and knelt down beside Matthew, I made myself really listen to him. I consciously chose obedience by letting go of my pride, by humbling myself and making myself listen to him. He was holding back tears and knew I was frustrated with him. But as I knelt down beside him and truly listened to him—to his *heart*—I could see that he was truly exhausted from no sleep the night before and a long day at school. So I told him I knew he was tired and that he was doing a great job. I gave him a hug, said I was sorry, and made him a deal that I would help push the mower and together we would finish the lawn. He even cried because he truly wanted to finish it by himself, but his body was just too tired. I was under conviction as I heard his cry. His frustration came from not being able to please us by doing what we asked the way we asked him. So I said I was sorry for my attitude and not listening to him, and together as father and son we finished the yard. It was a joy to help him once I let go of my pride. Even in those short moments, I went into an unconscious obedience of serving my tired son. The sequence went like this:

1. **Unconscious pride and lack of listening**
2. **Conscious pride and lack of listening**
3. **Conscious humility and listening**
4. **Unconscious humility and listening**

Being a good father doesn't mean being perfect—that is impossible. It is allowing myself to be humbled enough for God (and my wife) to correct me if I am wrong, to show me if I am being disobedient in some way. The only way I can teach my children obedience to God is by myself being teachable and asking forgiveness when I mess up. Only through my submission to God was I able to look past my pride to truly listen to him.

If you notice, every example is found in the "I Am" section in the form of a lie, and we are learning to change those lies with the truth. As God showed me I was in the wrong, He also showed me how to own the truth. I didn't focus on the negative or the fact that I was prideful. I changed it to "I am humble in the Lord" and "I am listening to Matthew's needs." I am a good father! The "I Am" is again taking ownership of the truth and power of God as He teaches us how to live obedient lives, which ultimately is our love affair with Jesus Christ.

So now comes the moment of truth! Once you realize that eating that double cheeseburger and super-sized order of fries every day for lunch is unhealthy, what are you going to do about it? Are you going to consciously choose to poison your body every day, or are you going to break those destructive behaviors and actions and make them obedient to Christ by eating healthy food? No, a cheeseburger once in a while is not disobedience, but living your life by throwing caution to the wind and doing whatever you want, whenever you want, certainly is! God wants all of us healthy, plain and simple. That doesn't mean being obsessive-compulsive. It does mean being healthy. As God shows you the root of your unhealthy behavior, what would it look like?

Remember: The goal of *Courage to Change* is for you to grow daily in your love affair with Jesus Christ, thus giving birth to an obedient, healthy lifestyle in every area of your life, including your physical health. By practicing the TAP principle and owning God's truth through the "I Am," you will begin to live by these principles unconsciously. They will become habits and second nature and will reflect your love affair with Jesus. May freedom, victory, and peace flow from you abundantly!

For Reflection:

Pinpoint some areas in your life where perfectionism is at work.

_____

_____

Combat those perfectionist lies with the truth.

_____

_____

What does it mean that "Christ's perfection is good enough for God"?

_____

_____

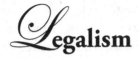egalism

*"The reign of terror present in the Body of Christ that wrongfully projects
the wrath, anger, and judgment of God on people"*

As you are learning about discipline and obedience, you must be aware of a serious problem present in the body of Christ. Let me begin with the story of Jo Anne.

An Epidemic: Legalism

I met Jo Anne, a woman in her early 50s, while personal training in Arlington, Texas. Within five minutes of meeting her, I could see that something was stealing her joy. She was whipped up and beaten down and didn't know why. Her teary eyes told me that she was longing for help. She was physically tired and weak and sometimes ached from head to toe. She told me that at some point she had lost her motivation and the will to be physically healthy and active. I asked her what was the source of her motivation, but I could sense that any talk of spirituality and God was a touchy subject.

As we stood there in the gym talking, it was as though a bubble enveloped us. I simply shared with her just how much God loved her, and as I did, the tears began to flow. She told me that she didn't know why she had felt compelled to pick the specific gym I was working at. Neither of us knew anything about each other, and I didn't purposely set up our meeting. It was a divine meeting—one that only God could set up. She couldn't believe she was listening to me talk about God as a loving God, her Father who would never leave her nor forsake her. She couldn't believe she was hearing that God was proud of her and that He longed to be in a relationship with her.

I took Jo Anne through my *Courage to Change* program and trained her for several months. In her, I saw firsthand the devastating effects of a very serious problem in our country. Jo Anne's had been raised under the reins of legalism, where children "were to be seen and not heard." She was taught an unhealthy fear of God and learned to tremble in His presence. She was told to beware of His judgment and expect His wrath if she didn't abide by *every biblical principle perfectly.* People in her life used the word of God to abuse, control, and manipulate her. People who were supposed to be in a position of trust and protection used their authority or position to silence her and control her to the point of destroying her confidence and ability to make decisions on her own. Decisions were made for her. She didn't have a voice. Only the people over her had a voice—people who called themselves her "spiritual authority," people in her family and church.

I remember so vividly how Jo Anne asked me if I was telling her the truth. She pleaded with me as she said, "Are you being serious? God really loves me and isn't disappointed in me? *He* really wants *me* in *His* life? He really wants me to talk to Him like a *friend* and to tell Him everything, even the things I struggle with?" She was overwhelmed to find out that what she hoped for throughout her whole life was true—that God did love her and was proud of her. God wasn't going to strike her dead if she crossed the street wrong. All her life she had wanted to have a relationship with God, but all she had been taught was judgment, wrath, and fear of God. She was never taught the love and gentleness of God, which was the entire reason Christ died for her. It is Christ who perfects her imperfections by covering her with Him (Colossians 3:3). Over the course of the few months we worked together, she lost 20 pounds, forgave the people who had spiritually abused her, and excitedly found herself a church. She attended one or two times every week, continued to journal, received a new confidence and voice from God, and was set free from her legalistic past. She was free!

Jesus said it himself, **"It is not the healthy that need a doctor, but the sick. But go and learn what this means: I desire mercy, not sacrifice. For I have not come to call the righteous, but sinners"** (Matthew 9:12–13). Every one of us sins or messes up from time to time, and that is why Christ came to us. He knew there would be a Bill or a Steve, a Suzie or a Debra, who was afraid, alone, lost, and craving forgiveness. He knew there would be a Joel, a Barbara, a Bonito or Delia, an Achmed, or an Achim who at times would fail to make the right choices and would long for forgiveness. It is our heart that yearns for the grace, mercy, and forgiveness that comes with Christ. Oh how beautiful He is!

I have dealt with some of this legalistic behavior myself. A while back, I became part owner of a fitness facility in Dallas, Texas. I knew that my business partner was a little rough around the edges, but as time went by his true colors came shining through. He was so afraid of losing control that he made life a sort of hell by controlling everything and everyone around him. The sad part was that he used scripture to justify his actions. While we worked on the business, he offered to help me with some formatting of an earler version of this very book. He didn't just offer help, he immediately tried taking control of it, which I stopped. He openly admitted that he had an agenda of controlling the rights to my book from the very beginning and even told me that if I didn't submit to his authority as the CEO, I would bring the judgment of God upon myself. He projected God's wrath on me by using Romans 13:1–2: **"Everyone must submit himself to the governing authorities, for there is no authority except that which God has established. The authorities that exist have been established by God. Consequently, he who rebels against the authority is rebelling against what God has instituted, and those who do so will bring judgment on themselves."**

If anyone had an individual thought or idea, he took it as rebellion against his authority. He would then reprimand and ridicule the person by pulling out scripture that he felt justified his anger. Romans 13:3–5 is an example of how he inflated himself and justified his anger and projection of God's wrath and judgment: **"For rulers hold no terror for those who do right, but for those who do wrong. Do you want to be free from fear of the one in authority? Then do what is right and he will commend you. For he is God's servant to do you good. But if you do wrong, be afraid, for he does not bear the sword for nothing. He is God's servant, an agent of wrath to bring punishment on the wrongdoer. Therefore, it is necessary to submit to the authorities, not only because of possible punishment but also because of conscience."**

Because, as the CEO, he was an employer, he literally thought he was an "agent of wrath to bring punishment on the wrongdoer"—his own employees and partner who didn't submit to his every command. When I told him I had a contact with a publisher, he told me I would fail and was in fact *a failure* without him. He would spend hours praying with clients and writing devotionals in his office then come out and cuss up a storm and project the judgment and wrath of God on his employees if they didn't "submit to his authority."

When I told him that I wasn't going to put up with his abuse and control any longer, he pulled out more scripture stating that a servant is subject to his master, even when the master is abusive. He literally saw himself as my "master." I owned 49% of the company and was a chief officer. Unbelievable! He led by fear, anger, and control. This behavior is not only ungodly but sick.

It was so bizarre that I actually questioned myself. I didn't want to believe someone was capable of using the beautiful word of God to control and manipulate me or anyone else. He knew how much I loved God and actually used that as he twisted the scriptures to his own advantage. The scary part was that I actually allowed him to control me for a while. I just didn't want to believe what he was doing. I didn't think it was possible. My emotions were all over the place. I felt trapped and paralyzed, just as he wanted me to. Once I realized and accepted what was happening, I got out of Dodge. My wife Silesia was instrumental in helping me see the truth of this behavior as I went through it. Our spirits are much too precious and important to God for us to stay in that kind of "reign of terror" day in and day out. I wonder how many other companies and even churches out there are run this way. It is wrong and needs to stop!

> **God absolutely sets up authority in business, homes, government, and the church, but it does not give any person a license to abuse, control, manipulate, and project the judgment of God on you!**

Legalism goes against the very nature of Christ. People who think that being an ambassador of Christ means controlling and projecting the wrath of God on people are wrong! They see themselves and their authority as a way to rule others. They take the word "govern" to mean a position of power that gives them permission to rule. The reason this goes against the very nature of Christ is because Jesus himself didn't come to rule or be served. *He came to serve!*

> **"Jesus called them together and said, 'You know that the rulers of the Gentiles lord it over them, and their high officials exercise authority over them. Not so with you. Instead, whoever wants to become great among you must be your servant, and whoever wants to be first must be your slave just as the Son of Man did not come to be served, but to serve, and to give his life as a ransom for many.'"** (Matthew 20:25–28)

This is called **servitude leadership.** Whoever is in a position of authority and governs others has a greater responsibility to serve, not to rule! Those in authority in business, the home, church, and government are slaves to those they govern, meaning that *they* are the servants. Those in authority must display humility, compassion, and empathy. All of us who love Jesus are called to live this way. I don't rule over my employees or my clients. I serve them. I don't rule over my wife and children as the head of the house. I have the greatest responsibility to serve in my family. I am not only my family's physical protector but their spiritual covering as well. Of course, my wife is covered by Jesus, but I have a responsibility to protect her, to keep her vulnerable heart safe. Silesia does an amazing job of protecting my heart as well. Being a servant leader is beautiful. It is an honor and makes God happy!

Many of you have been brought up in legalism or spiritual abuse. My heart breaks when I find out how people have turned their backs on God or the church because of someone else's perverted teachings and idiocy. If any of you have been brought up with, or are in some way being abused with this kind of behavior, first know that it is wrong. God does love you even when you make mistakes. His promise to you is to never leave you nor forsake you. You are His child, His son or daughter, and He will always be there for you and love you.

Silesia's Testimony

At this time my amazing wife Silesia is going to share with you her story of how she has overcome the spiritual abuse of legalism and how it affects your body and ability to take care of yourself. Every time I listen to her express her love and faith in God, I fall in love with her all over again—to say nothing of my love for God, too! I hope her beautiful heart touches you as it has touched me and all who have met her.

> From Silesia:
> I remember the Sunday morning as if it happened yesterday. My daughter Shelby had been begging me to go and visit a church we had attended before we moved a few years before. It had been a long time since we had been there and I had not stayed in touch. My soul was dying. I was in an abusive marriage (before Brian) and I was blaming God. I knew the ugly state of my heart. So we visited the church, and while there, I was approached by three different women. One even had tears in her eyes as she asked me how I was. She had been thinking of me and praying for me. That's what each of the women said. As I sat in the service reminding God of my frustration with my life and holding back tears from the love those special ladies bestowed on me, God gently spoke to my heart: "I will pursue you with my love." "Me?" I thought. I didn't deserve His love—I knew the sad state of my heart and that I had been blaming Him for other people's actions. It was a new concept for me to accept that God pursues me. If I would but open the eyes of my heart, He would romance me as only the author of romance could.
>
> I was raised in the church and I married a man I met in church. So how could the fact that God loved me seem like such a foreign concept? The answer is this: legalism, or put another way, *religious abuse.* I know that it must absolutely break God's heart that so many wounded people have sustained their injuries through church members and church leaders. Have you had God's judgment proclaimed on you? Have people used God's laws and principles to manipulate and harm you?
>
> I have not often spoken of the abuse I experienced growing up. "Loyalty" to the family has paralyzed my voice for too long. As I share specific situations, even now I have to overcome the fear that some of you will think it is far too

bizarre to be true. I have asked God and Brian if there are people who can relate to what I have survived. It seems to me that abuse in the church is a well-kept secret, at least it was in my family.

I don't recall having too many bad experiences as a little girl. But in my teens things changed. My dad was a preacher in the small town where I grew up. Before becoming a preacher, Dad had spent 20 years in the army. He served many tours in Vietnam and was a hero in many ways. But there was a side of my father that church members never saw. My dad was very controlling and very, very angry. I was never quite sure what set him off, but oh what I would do to try to avoid the explosion. I was an overachiever in school. I remember in high school handing my straight-A report card to my dad. I was really proud of my effort and hard work. He looked at it and said, "Why aren't these A-pluses?" I giggled, thinking he was joking. He wasn't. He was completely serious. On another occasion I remember him lunging at me and yelling at the top of his lungs. I was so scared because I thought he was going to hit me that time. I can still hear my voice, "Don't hit me, Daddy!" I cringed in terror. I could never agree and apologize fast enough to satisfy him.

My mother always assumed the role of bystander. Never once did she ever stand up for us or stop him. I always assumed she was scared of him, too, until one day she blamed dad's fit of rage on me saying, "You invited Satan into our home! Your father's anger is *your* fault!"

I carried so much guilt and shame. Keeping the "happy Christian family" façade alive took a lot of energy. Hiding these secrets was preparation for the abusive marriage I stayed in for well over a decade. My parents were idolized in the church. My father was the minister for the police station, and my bruises were never physical. Who could I turn to for help? I once saw my dad throw my brother onto the hood of the car. Another time I remember him screaming at me until I blacked out and could hear nothing. Suicide seemed like my only option for escape...until a very soft-spoken college guy entered the picture promising me love.

So I ran away and got married—only to find I had married a much "quieter" version of control and anger. Once again he was a master of disguise, always keeping up appearances for church members. So many times, and for such a long time, I believed that if I were a better daughter, or a better wife, these men wouldn't be so mad and God wouldn't be so disappointed in me. After all, it was "in God's name" that they behaved this way! My eyes tear up even now as I remember the painful place where I dwelled. I was convinced that there was something so wrong with me and that this anger was the effect I had on men.

My dad, suspecting that I was planning to get married to escape, told me gently one morning that God himself had told him that if I got married against his will, I would never be able to have children. I believed this to be true. I thought my dad had a direct connection to God. Many times he would tell me, "God tells me when you are doing something you aren't supposed to, so don't think you can get away with anything!" I even overheard my parents praying that God would just kill me rather than let me get married.

Fear! Fear! Fear! I was afraid of my parents, afraid of my husband, afraid of God, afraid of life. Death truly seemed so comforting. Even in my late 30s, as I was weeks away from marrying the godly man of my dreams, Brian, one family member said that since I was divorced and single and my father was deceased, he was the authority in my life and that Brian had no biblical right to protect me until we are married. He called my home 30 times one evening harassing me. Another family member still calls and leaves me messages stating that my children and I are not protected by God and that I have once again invited Satan into my home. This is crazy behavior, and it is never what God desires for our lives. It goes against His very character. I am so confident of His love for me, my children, and even my abusive family.

I now know to the core of my being that even though I am not perfect, God is not disappointed and ashamed of me. He is so in love with me. He is faithful and never intended for His word to be a weapon of destruction. My friend, if you have endured shaming, blame, and pain at the hands of churchgoing people, please know that God's very big arms are longing to embrace and sustain you. The difficult things in your life are not punishment. In fact, many of the difficult things in your life are the result of you being exactly where God wants you to be. You do not have to "measure up" to deserve the love and grace of God in your life. He is so in love with you. He doesn't love you because of what you do for Him. When your children were born, did you give birth to them so they could help with chores? No, it is about the relationship. God doesn't love you for what you do or don't do. It is truly about an unconditional love, the likes of which I had never experienced. He is absolutely head over heals in love with you!!!

So how does legalism affect your physical health? The root of legalism is fear, not love; fear of disappointing God or people. When I am afraid and focused on trying not to make a mistake, it hinders me from loving and living. For me, living in controlling and abusive relationships was so draining that I had no desire to take care of myself. Something amazing that I have seen happen for my clients as well as myself is this: As I got physically stronger through my workouts, my voice became strengthened and empowered. I have seen clients begin to exercise and thus plant a seed that blossomed into amazing, healthy changes—some have started their own businesses and were empowered to get out of unhealthy relationships. And it started with exercise. I have often said that **exercise trains you for life.** This is so true because stress and grief produce so many harmful chemicals in our bodies, and exercise helps us rid our bodies of these toxins. Every day that you invest in your health truly is training for life.

In the last few years of my dad's life, we experienced much healing and restoration in our relationship. His death was quite difficult, and for the first time, my workouts took a drastic change. Rather than weight training, I focused more on relaxation and stretching in the form of yoga (not of Eastern influence) and pilates, which helped calm my being. I knew my mind, body, and spirit had been heavily taxed with his death coming so suddenly after a painful divorce. There were months of shaking and waking up with panic attack symptoms. I was gentle with my body as it recovered and healed. I kept telling myself that the years of working out would really pay off now as my body was being pushed to the extreme.

As you find the *Courage to Change* your health, I want to encourage you on the days that seem too hard to work out to visualize yourself training for life. Allow your workouts the flexibility to fit into your life. As a single mom after my divorce, many of my workouts were at the park with my children. Racing them and playing with them not only got my workout done, but also set an example to them of health and fitness. Be good to your "being"; be patient and kind. If you are struggling to be set free from an unhealthy relationship or abuse of some kind, remember to surround yourself with people who desire you to be healthy and who encourage you to make good, healthy choices. The Bible tells us that we reap what we sow: **"Remember this: Whoever sows sparingly will also reap sparingly, and whoever sows generously will also reap generously. Each man should give what he has decided in his heart to give, not reluctantly or under compulsion, for God loves a cheerful giver"** (2 Corinthians 9:6–7). I want to challenge you today to make baby steps of planting seeds into your health and the health of your loved ones. Be ready for the miracle of "YOU" to blossom!

—Love, Silesia

Take Heart: Forgive and Move On

Silesia and I don't blame anyone for his or her actions. There is no resentment or anger. We are free from this behavior because we have forgiven and recognize the truth of a God who pursues us every moment with love, gentleness, and grace, not with wrath, fear, and domination through people. He lets us know when we mess up, but as a proud Father He teaches us with His loving hands. Through eyes of love, He watches over us and keeps us on track and in alignment with Him as much as possible. Through Jesus Christ we are healed and free to live our lives *not* by the law but by grace, which enables us to obey Him with joy, honor, respect, and awe. If you have been hurt by legalism, please don't turn your back on the church as a whole. We encourage all of you to find yourself a grace-full church in which you can grow and flourish and be fed the richness of God's love and grace. We believe in the church, God's principles, laws, and authority, and in the importance of obedience. They are all beautiful if we learn them through Christ.

My friends, breaking free from religious abuse and every other kind of abuse takes effort and time. You will heal. The action you take with exercise and good nutrition is a crucial factor in learning to be confident in your faith and discovering that you have a voice that counts! Remember, God's most basic gift to you is your life. Your most basic gift back to Him is your health. Taking care of yourself won't make God love you any more, and not taking care of yourself won't make God love you any less. Taking care of yourself is simply a physical love letter (a love note from *you* to God) you write to God daily that tells Him, **"Thank you for my life!"**

For Reflection:

Has there been a time in your life when you were on the giving or receiving end of religious or spiritual abuse? Describe the experience and its effects.

_____

_____

Are there any trappings of a legalist upbringing or experience you need to forgive and get over? Explain.

_____

_____

If so, what action will you take to forgive and move on and walk in grace and Christian liberty?

_____

_____

STRESS!

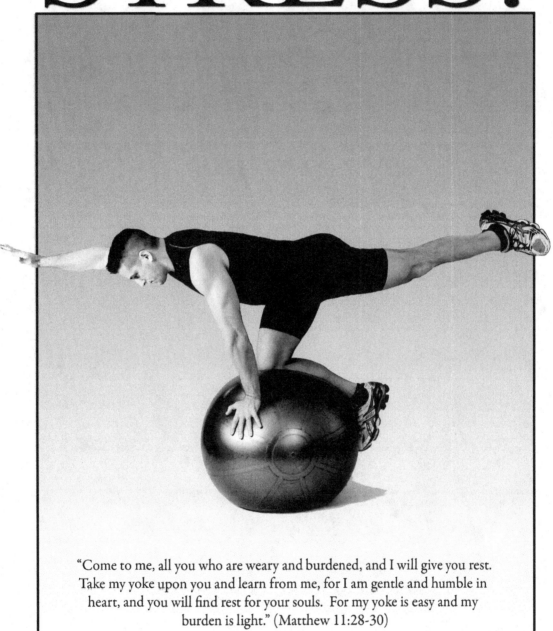

"Come to me, all you who are weary and burdened, and I will give you rest.
Take my yoke upon you and learn from me, for I am gentle and humble in
heart, and you will find rest for your souls. For my yoke is easy and my
burden is light." (Matthew 11:28-30)

WEEK FIVE

tress

The circumstances of everyday life are rough. Has a traffic jam ever pushed you beyond the limit of what you could handle? What about the roar of loud engines and the blinding red of brake lights from all the cars endlessly trying to get somewhere? Or what about the huge construction machines plowing up the earth and making horrible noises and making it impossible to drive? Then there are the kids screaming at each other, thousands of horns honking, tempers flaring, murder reports and bombings on the news, planes and helicopters flying overhead, the sirens of police cars and ambulances forging through the traffic, bills to pay, dogs barking, car alarms beeping, cell phones ringing, anger, hatred, fear . . . *when does it all stop?*

It doesn't!

But you can change how you deal with it all! Stress can be both good and bad. *Eustress* is stress that helps prepare us for something. An example of eustress is eagerly anticipating or eagerly awaiting a result we are working for. Eustress is so-called "good" or healthy (*eu*) stress. But when you find yourself having way too many things happening at the same time, or turn your focus off of God, *eustress* can easily turn into *distress.*

Distress is the number one cause of illness and death. Some people say that obesity, poor nutrition, and/or smoking is the number one cause. Take your pick—they all cause distress to the body, the mind, and the emotions of everyone who interacts directly or indirectly with distressed people. There are thousands of stressors in the world. Some may surprise you. Children screaming may not be a violation of your spirit, but any anger, impatience, and intolerance toward them would be. Car alarms beeping and cell phones ringing may not be, but anytime you turn your eyes away from Christ and onto your circumstances you engage in distress because the world is a stressed-out place.

In this section we will be considering authority, godly principles, laws, and obedience. As we do, please remember what we said in the previous section on legalism. Please don't let these terms scare you as we talk about them. When used and practiced correctly and in their proper contexts, they are for your protection and based on love, not on control, abuse, or manipulation. Whether in business, government, home, or even church, when people use their position of authority to control, abuse, or manipulate you, they are not operating from the true standard and character that God has set in place. So remember that God gives us principles to live by because He loves us—as a loving Father loves His children!

Distress can be thought of as simply taking your focus off of God and putting it on your circumstances, either directly or indirectly.

Focusing on your circumstances indirectly is allowing the world around you to affect you. Focusing on your circumstances directly is being disobedient. Any time you are out of alignment with God, distress of some kind will result. Using the example of road rage, how many times have you been stressed out because others around you were cutting you off and flying by you? Better yet, how many times have you felt stressed out because you were late and speeding to get somewhere and you were the one doing the cutting? The reason you feel stressed is because you are focused on your circumstances (being late and probably being mad at yourself) and as a result, by speeding, you are breaking the law that your governing authorities have established for your protection. The clincher is that those same governing authorities were originally established by God, and we all are commanded to submit to them.

> **"Everyone must submit himself to the governing authorities, for there is no authority except that which God has established. The authorities that exist have been established by God. Consequently, he who rebels against the authority is rebelling against what God has instituted, and those who do so will bring judgment on themselves. For rulers hold no terror for those who do right, but for those who do wrong. Do you want to be free from fear of the one in authority? Then do what is right and he will commend you."** (Romans 13:1–3)

As Paul stated here in Romans, distress is a form of rebellion. Come on, we all have rebelled by speeding at one time or another! But as you obey the law and drive the speed limit, your focus remains on God and His principles and established laws, which keeps you far removed from stress and harm. Tying in this example with the "I Am" declaration and TAP principle will illustrate the importance of this kind of spiritual alignment:

	Believed lie	I change my belief to:
Thought→	I am late and impatient	I am patient in my lateness ☺
Attitude→	I am angry	I am peaceful, I am gentle, I am kind
Performance→	I am speeding	I am submitting to my governing authorities and God by driving the speed limit.

This and the following scenario are two of thousands of stressful situations. Understanding the difference between thoughts, attitudes, and performances is important while learning to retrain or prepare your mind for action.

God has also established a law of good health when he tells you **"to offer your bodies as living sacrifices, holy and pleasing to God—this is your spiritual act of worship"** (Romans 12:1) and **"Do you not know that your body is a temple of the Holy Spirit, who is in you, whom you have received from God? You are not your own; you were bought at a price. Therefore, honor God with your body"** (1 Corinthians 6:19–20).

Not taking care of the amazing body God gave you with exercise and good nutrition is a violation of your spirit. For after all, "You are not your own. You were bought at a price." And again this violation causes stress. Does this mean never eating a cheeseburger again? Absolutely not! It applies to constant overeating, gluttonous behavior, and a sedentary lifestyle. Tying in this example with the "I Am" and TAP is as follows:

		Believed lie	I change my belief to:
Thought→		I am fat, repulsive and ugly	I am beautiful, I am radiant, I am handsome, I am lovely, I am elegant
Attitude→		I am insecure	I am secure in the Lord
Performance→		I am not taking care of myself physically	I am taking care of myself daily with good nutrition and exercise

Once you have identified what is stressing you out, all three of these must be changed to overcome and conquer it. You can do it!

If even one of these is out of alignment, it is a violation of your spirit and will cause distress and negative results. Even if you change the thought of "I am ugly" to "I am beautiful or handsome," it will not produce the results you want if your attitude is still insecure. All three must be changed.

As I stated earlier, even if you change your actions, you can still be controlled through your thoughts and attitude. Fear and resentment can riddle you even though you have changed the actions. How many times have you begun an exercise and nutrition program only to find yourself hit with a barrage of thoughts of insecurity, inability, weakness, doubt, and hopelessness? How many times has it become a stressor in your life and ultimately made you quit? There is no shame. There is no guilt. *But it is time to change!*

Addressing the Cause—Not Just the Symptoms—of Stress

Most sickness is caused by stress of some kind. Our society tells us that exercise reduces stress, which is only partly true. Exercise and good nutrition do battle stress mainly by alleviating the *symptoms* of stress rather than its *causes,* which need to be addressed for real stress-relief to occur. A client in Arlington, Texas came to me because he wanted an exercise program to help him reduce his stress levels. He was on blood pressure medication for the stress and had a very busy, high-profile, demanding career. He asked me to design a program for him as well as make other suggestions for things he could do to reduce his stress. He honestly thought that exercise and other "doingness" would help solve his stress issues. My response was this:

If you base your health on "doingness" while taking care of your stress, you will "DO" yourself to death!

157

If you engage in exercise "doingness", it will become just another stressor in your life, like everything else. Don't deal with your stress by your "doingness." Sure, exercise helps with the symptoms of stress but it does not address the *cause* of stress. After exercise your body releases a hormone called relactin, which gives you a sort of euphoric feeling and relaxes you. It is your body's own muscle relaxant. But if you exercise to keep dealing with the symptoms of your stress without getting at its cause, then you never truly move forward because whatever is causing you to get down, tired, depressed, and agitated is still there. All you end up doing is continuing to throw water on the flames instead of putting out the fire at the source.

As you exercise and reap the benefits of a stronger yet more relaxed body, how do you battle the cause of stress? It all goes back to God. What my client didn't realize was that his high-profile job had been entrusted to him because of his amazing gifts and his ability to lead in his chosen profession. The same God who had given him that career position and the gifts to be great in it would also give him everything he needed to handle the responsibilities that went with it.

Once he realized that he could not deal with the cause of his stress by his "doingness" but only by relying on the love and grace of God, he felt a release. I could see his entire body let go of an amazing weight, a heaviness slowly driving him into the ground. I told him to eat right, exercise to be healthy, and honor God but not to do it as the means to handle all of his stress. Exercise has its purpose and benefits, but it is still just exercise, which, compared to the amazing love and peace found in Christ, is nothing. This is why when we put all of our motivation in fitness instead of God, we burn out and get the yo-yo syndrome over and over again instead of being consistent with our health for the rest of our lives. *So let exercise help deal with the flames of the fire, but let God put the fire out completely.* That way, exercise can become an enjoyable experience instead of always just a weapon to deal with something negative.

I used to play the piano whenever I was stressed out or hurting. Sometimes I still do. But after a few years I realized that I associated the piano with hurt, depressed emotions, and therapy. It was very hard for me to play the piano when I was in a good mood because my inspiration (i.e., suffering) wasn't there. So I taught myself to let my other emotions of peace and joy and happiness bring forth the same beautiful music as I did before. Now I can play the piano for a 30-minute session and experience just about the whole range of emotions, not just the painful ones. In the same way, there is a process of learning and disciplining yourself to develop a love for exercise, not just to take care of the stress but to become such a part of your day that you feel that something is missing when you don't get it. And much like playing the piano, exercise is simply another way of expressing yourself. Both require physical action and discipline and require you to honor the gifts God has given you. So be an instrument and use your body to play a song for God every time you breathe and sweat and feel your muscles burn as you work them. He is the greatest audience you will ever play for.

Why all this talk about stress?

Whenever your spirit is violated, your body has automatic physiological responses to that stress. Your body is an emotional garbage disposal. When you focus on your circumstances and not God, the physiological response is a release of a hormone called cortisol, which feeds on muscle tissue. It is the same hormone that gets released into your bloodstream when you are sick, making it very difficult for your body to recover and repair itself. If you are exercising and breaking your muscles down to be rebuilt stronger but your body can't repair them, you stay in a constant state of breakdown. This distress also causes you to restrict your breathing and inhibits your body's ability to provide oxygen-rich blood to the many organs systems and processes of your body.

Your body cannot even digest healthy food when you are stressed because your digestive system goes haywire due to the release of stress-related hormones and acids in your body. Even if you are diligent with your exercise and eat right, stress of any kind will dramatically affect your ability to lose weight and be physically healthy because your body stores that stress in the form of poisons and toxins. Remember: Every single thing you do in life, good or bad, brings a physiological response. Isn't it interesting that when you exercise your body releases relactin, the relaxation hormone? God gave you everything you need, even built-in muscle-relaxing hormones that are only released as a reward for doing physical exercise.

In your *Life Application Journal,* you will start each day with victory by tapping into God by writing positive life-changing affirmations as validated with God's word in the Bible. This will help you focus on God throughout the day and give your body the healing, stress-free environment it needs to get healthy.

For Reflection:

Are there some activities in your life that you do to "cope with stress" that address only the symptoms and not the cause of the stress?

_____

_____

As you think about the stress in your life, move beyond the symptoms to the causes? What can you do to address the causes rather than just the symptoms? What changes do you need to make?

_____

_____

Sleep and Relaxation

Being healthy does not simply mean exercising all the time or adhering perfectly to your nutrition plan. Besides exercise and good nutrition, relaxation also plays a critical role in your health. Without it, you lack concentration and energy, feel nervous and uptight, develop sleep disorders, and lose the ability to express yourself.

There is a big difference between sleep and relaxation. One must be conscious to relax. If you go to bed without first relaxing, you will sleep restlessly and wake up in the morning with the same stress you went to bed with. When you sleep, your body is busy healing itself and charging you up physically and mentally for the next day. So don't rely on sleep to relax you. If you burden your sleep center with relaxation, it will overload and cause you to lose sleep. When this happens, you are neither relaxed nor properly rested. The average person should sleep a minimum of six hours per night and eight hours is optimal—but only *after* attaining a proper state of relaxation. **"Do not let the sun go down while you are still angry"** (Ephesians 4:26). This scripture also applies to stress of any kind. Deal with it before your head hits the pillow, and watch as your sleep becomes much more restful.

> **"Come to me, all you who are weary and burdened, and I will give you rest. Take my yoke upon you and learn from me, for I am gentle and humble in heart, and you will find rest for your souls. For my yoke is easy and my burden is light."** (Matthew 11:28–30)

God tells us to come to Him with our burdens. He promises that when we do He will give us "rest for our souls." He fulfills this promise by giving us both internal rest and physical rest and relaxation because they are all interconnected. Learning to relax is part of the process of bettering yourself. To relax is to control your emotions and learn how to control or manipulate the environment around you to exemplify more of God's love and grace. By going out of your way to relax, you become in tune with yourself, because you are taking the time to be closer to God. Though it is important to excuse yourself from your daily routine to relax, it is more important to learn to relax while doing your everyday activities. It is in your everyday activities that He tells you, **"Come to me, all you who are weary and burdened."** This means work, family, exercise, everything!

Music...Charms to Soothe the Savage Breast (and Relax You!)

Music is a beautiful tool for relaxing because it helps you enter into the Holy Spirit wherever you are. Below is a list of musical pieces that are quite soothing and stimulating. Since nature is such a part of all of us, many of the artists I have selected have integrated instrumental music with the sounds of nature:

- Enya
- Classical
- Yanni
- Gospel
- John Tesh
- Contemporary Christian
- *LifeScapes*
- George Winston
- NatureQuest
- Mannheim Steamroller
- *Echoes of Nature*
- John Williams
- David Lanz
- Kenny G
- Danny Wright
- Billy Joe Walker
- *The Enchanted Garden*
- Ed Van Fleet

Barnes and Noble, Blockbuster Music, Target, and many other retailers offer different varieties of music. Look around and find the type of music that moves you. You will know when it happens. The right kind of music fills you up inside, relinquishes hidden stresses you do not want, and inspires you.

The right kind of music will stimulate and inspire you from the inside out and also enhance your physical performance during exercise. By stimulating music I am not talking about loud, obnoxious music with someone screaming profanity at you. That kind of music squelches your spirit. I am talking about music that brings out your passion and stimulates your spirit.

Your body is stimulated and/or programmed by what you let enter you. Your mind must be set or programmed for action first, then the body will follow during whatever activity you want to perform. Just as the praise portion of your church service helps you enter into and receive the word from your pastor or priest, the same is true with any kind of physical performance.

Listening to instrumental, classical, or other passionate music before an event programs your mind and emotions for action because of its direct impact on your spirit. This is where true strength comes from. Something loud and obnoxious will overstimulate you and won't last. The idea is to relax your body to enable it to perform optimally without using up any unnecessary energy. Whether at work or getting ready to work out, music is a great way to keep your body relaxed and passionately inspired to perform.

> **"The LORD is my strength and my shield; my heart trusts in him, and I am helped. My heart leaps for joy and I will give thanks to him in song."**
> (Psalms 27:7)

If you find yourself feeling stressed, here are a few things you must do. First, ask yourself what is causing your distress. Sometimes it is obvious, and sometimes it may take a while to figure out.

Once you have figured out why you are stressed, don't stop there. The biggest problem most people face is that once they have the answer they don't do anything with it. You must take action and solve the problem as best you can. Many times the cause of stress will be very simple. During my first job in the health industry, I found that having a disorganized desk made me stressed. It showed up in the form of a headache. So I would take two minutes to organize the desk and I would find myself perfectly OK later on, with no headache.

My favorite commercial of all time shows a little boy about six years old sitting on his front steps with a tray on his lap. On his tray he has a giant glass of milk and a can of Hershey's chocolate syrup. He proceeds to open the can of chocolate syrup and begins to pour it into the glass of milk. To his dismay, the can is just about empty and only a little is dripping out. So he thinks a moment. At this point he still hasn't said a word. As if an epiphany strikes his mind, he sets the can of chocolate syrup down. He picks up the glass of milk and begins pouring the milk into the can of chocolate syrup. Once he is finished pouring, he puts the lid on the can and confidently shakes it up. He then pops the lid off and pours the most perfect glass of chocolate milk you have ever seen. Then he takes a big sip of it and looks up with a chocolaty grin and says, "If there is one thing in life my father has always taught me, there are no problems in life, only solutions!" I have done my best to live by this principle. It has helped tremendously in virtually every area of my life and has helped me better deal with stress. *Change your thinking to solution-solving instead of problem-solving!*

Learning to relax involves not only your ability to practice positive thinking and find solutions to problems, but also your ability to express emotions. Each of you has beautiful emotions just waiting to be released. That means you too, guys! Perhaps these feelings are bottled up inside because of past pain, egotism, and insecurity, or maybe you have never taken steps to learn how to express yourself. Everything you do, in one form or another, is an expression of yourself. The way you walk demonstrates confidence, or a lack thereof; the way you talk suggests enthusiasm, or a lack thereof; and the way you smile demonstrates your personality. Exercise, eating, laughing, crying, breathing, and loving are all common forms of expression. Everything we do matters to us, and everything we do has an impact in some way on someone else.

We observe people every day. What does it mean to observe someone or something? Observing means seeing the *expressions* of whatever it is we are looking at. We have choices all the time. Does a child always walk on the sidewalk? No! The child chooses to walk on the curb or in the grass, balances on some landscape timbers, or walks with arms out like wings in take-off position. **Is that childish, or is that the essence of life?** We get so caught up in being adults that we forget to use our imaginations. We forget how to express ourselves. And then we wonder why over 60% of all marriages end in divorce! Well, I'll tell you something—**if more adults would walk on the curb or in the grass, balance on landscape timbers, or hold their arms up for take-off, there would be less divorce in the world! Let yourself go once in a while. Invite yourself to come out and play! Open your hearts and minds to one another, and be healthy.**

The Three Elements of Relaxation

Three main elements are needed to achieve relaxation: (1) feeling, (2) expression, and (3) imagination. Often we get so focused on how other people are feeling that we do not take the time to actually experience our own feelings. Learn to be more observant and open to the things around you. Don't just acknowledge that a bird is chirping; listen carefully and try to figure out what it is saying. Whistle back if you want to. Come on guys, remember my story in chapter one? If a manly-man body builder dude in college (me) could do it, so can you! By actually listening to the bird, you are allowing yourself to feel and experience an incredible emotion based on a simple sound. This will make you a better listener altogether, something we all need! By whistling back to the bird you involve yourself both in feeling and expression. Remember: How you choose to express yourself is very important. Do you whistle shyly or aggressively? The way you whistle to the bird also depends on how the bird is whistling. Whistling in a different tone or key may scare the bird away. Apply this concept to your home life. If someone is speaking to you and you do not listen carefully, you will not have the proper response and may even hurt that person's feelings. Like the bird, that person may fly away! So learn to express yourself, not just for other people but also for yourself.

Learning to express yourself is actually a gift you give yourself because it enhances your ability to feel. If you give yourself something, you feel good, right? Learn to play a musical instrument, sing in the shower, sing to your kids or your spouse, write poetry, or paint. **Forget about perfection and let yourself go. Get over yourself and have some fun please!**

Where does imagination come into all this? Like the child playing with a magic carpet or having tea with a princess, use your imagination to create your own heaven on earth—it is imaginary only if you allow it to be! Being secure enough in yourself to truly express your emotions and be imaginative both verbally and physically takes time. It is a process—a journey for you to enjoy! Remember that **learning is the journey and knowledge is your destination!** Letting go means that you are completely secure in yourself in a vulnerable situation. Being vulnerable means leaving yourself open to the good and to the bad simultaneously. This is the essence of having control of your life!

While learning to take care of yourself, engage in creative activities. Learn to play the piano, write a book, or compose poetry for your spouse or a loved one. Take voice lessons, dance lessons, painting classes, woodworking classes, or even sculpture classes. TAP into the amazing gifts God has given you to express yourself.

Leslie, a 43-year-old female in Denver, came to me in 1999 ready to make a serious change in her life. She had a high-profile, high-stress corporate job with tremendous responsibility and a heavy workload. She was tired, worn-out, and out of shape and she desperately wanted help. So we went to work. I gave her a two- to three-hour consultation, which covered the original content of the *Courage to Change* program. In that power-packed session we covered nutrition, cardio, weight training, and behavior. We then began training two times per week. I trained her and her husband separately once per week and together as a couple once per week.

Leslie had undergone extensive surgery on both knees and they ached throughout each day. Within nine weeks she had lost 25 pounds and looked amazing. Over the course of a year of training with me, she was able to perform a perfect functional squat with 95 pounds on her shoulders. She could do this 20 times in three separate sets for a total of 60 repetitions. Remember, this is after having extensive knee surgery. Remember, too, that Leslie was a career woman "corporate type" not a professional athlete! She also took up woodworking as a hobby to stimulate her creative side. From scratch she built a very ornate dining room table for her home and took on many exciting projects. She did all this, mind you, while upholding the responsibilities of her high-end corporate job. Her husband retired, and the two of them enjoy their youthful health again. Her husband lost 30 pounds in 11 weeks, and both he and Leslie have kept the weight off. It was truly a joy for me to see their transformation from the inside out. Their humility in asking me for help and their committed hard work continues to inspire me to keep myself in amazing shape and to continue to strive for excellence in everything I do.

Seizing the Day in a Trying Time

Like you, I have experienced many stressful ordeals in my life. I would like to share a rather big one and how I dealt with it. During my youth (as now), I was blessed with a good family full of love and friendship. One thing I had to deal with was death. It seemed as though every time I turned around, someone died. By the time I graduated from high school, I thought I had seen enough, but it kept on coming. By my 21st birthday I had been to over 20 funerals. I once wrote a paper comparing myself to Hamlet. The similarities were scary. There I was in college not knowing who I was. I had all this emotion dammed up inside me. *What was the meaning of life? Why was I here? Why was I so passionate about everything I did?* Society told me I couldn't change the world and that I was foolish to try. All I could do was pick a major and stay in that track for the rest of my life. I became a bear to live with. I am not sure how my family stood me. I wasn't sure how to talk about these things and all of the death because they had to go through it, too. So I withdrew from my family and became a bitter person for a while.

I knew what the problem was, but I did not know how to accept it. All I knew was that I didn't know who I was, people were dropping like flies, and I was miserable! Though my family had always been very supportive and open, I wasn't open to them. Two main influences helped re-channel my negativity. The first was simply a movie that dealt with who I was as a person. The second was a poem. These two very simple things had a profound influence on my life. The movie was *Dead Poets Society* and it helped validate the passion I had inside of me. I sat enthralled throughout the movie and took in its philosophy: SEIZE THE DAY, BOYS! It made me realize that though I may not be able to change the "whole" world, I could certainly do my best to change a big chunk of it! To this day I am dedicated to the people of the world, people like you, and how I can possibly enrich your lives. Though *Dead Poets Society* is a secular movie, it spoke to my heart and validated in me the passion I had to help people.

A simple movie had a dramatic impact on how I perceived myself. But the death was still there. An aunt and uncle from different families had committed suicide. A cousin died of a drug overdose. Two friends committed suicide. Another cousin was murdered. It seems I was touched by every kind of death possible. I remember visiting my grandmother Cyrilla in the ICU. She had been in a coma for a while. Only half-conscious, she took my hands and gently rubbed my strong, very calloused hands across her lips. As she did this, she said over and over again, "So strong, so strong, so strong!" She died one day after my 20th birthday. Six months later my other grandmother suffered a heart attack after opening Christmas presents on Christmas Eve. I gave her CPR, but she didn't make it. Within another six months, my Aunt Barbara was found dead of a brain aneurysm.

All this left me in a state of despair. So one night about 2 a.m., after everyone was in bed, I took out some paper and a pencil and tried to figure everything out. I started by asking God and myself a question: "Must everything die?" Please notice that I started with a question that doesn't seem to get answered, but I kept asking anyway. I was frustrated, but I was desperate for an answer. After a while, a feeling came upon me. I started to see things more clearly. My pen kept writing, my emotions were spewing all over the paper, and I finally answered the question, "Must everything die?"

Must Everything Die?

I look out my window,
lay my weary head on its *pain*.
Leaves I see falling, down,
    down they fall.
I look away.
    Must everything die?

Birds dive, falling—down,
    down they fall!
But they do not die
    but again soar upward,
upward they fly!
Still, I look away.
    They will die someday,
    Must everything die?

Oh beautiful sunrise,
    tell me thou art weak,
    like the bird you fall each night
    but do not die!
    Will you die someday
like the bird?
    Should I look away?

I look out my window
lay my weary head on its *pain*.
My reflection I see sitting, there,
    there it sits!
    I look away.
    I will die someday.
    Must everything die?

As I look away
I now look about my life,

but there is more,
more than I to see,
as I stare at my life before me!
There are memories,
memories of those deceased, buried,
buried by their priests!
How can this be? They have died!
But the memories do not hide
they do indeed live on,
on they stride!

Again
I look out my window,
lay my calmed head on its *pane*,
and remember yesterday's leaves
and yesterday's birds that dove, down, down they dove!
See—they have not died
but live on inside me!

God gave me a heart to cherish
life—a soul to cherish
death—and a mind to record all that has happened!

My heart feeds the mind
these memories
so the soul can take them further!
And my home with its memories
and love is like a
mortal heaven!

Yes, we do die!
But are reborn as memories
and the most beautiful, intrinsic colors in heaven!

We are caterpillars in this world
while... life is but a cocoon
and heaven its butterfly!

I ask you to
look out your window
lay your weary head on its *pain*
and ask yourself,

Must everything die?

If you are wondering why I have included this story in my book on health, here's why: It is one of the great reasons I feel such a passion for helping people like you live healthy, happy, and productive lives. I have seen the alternative my whole life. The many deaths I mentioned happened prior to my writing that poem. Since writing it, I have also buried my father, father-in-law, brother Aaron, aunt Helen, and cousin Shelly. I have seen death of every kind. I have seen families, including my own, ripped apart by unforeseen events, unhealthy behaviors, and poor lifestyle choices. I could have let it harden my heart, but instead I dedicated my life to people like you who ask for help, who might not be able to find your joy on your own and get healthy.

Taking Stock

We are here on earth but a short time. Many things are out of our control, but so much *is* in our control. Let's all commit right now to look at the value of the life God has given us and cherish it with our healthy actions. Maybe you have heart disease or diabetes because you don't take care of yourself. Or maybe you have such a low self-worth that you are contemplating suicide, as did my aunt and uncle and friends. **Stop, don't do it! YOU ARE beautiful and loved! Do you have any idea *how much* you are loved? No amount of stress can keep you from the love of God! He is the pursuer of your soul even as you read this! He loves you so much! No amount of pain is too much for God to free you from! There is help and there is hope!**

If God could bring good to my life out of the death I have seen, He will bring good to your situation as well because He loves us both the same. We are both His children and He loves us equally. You are simply my brother or sister. We are family and belong to Jesus. With help you will get healthy physically, emotionally, mentally, and spiritually. You have the strength inside you, otherwise, you wouldn't be reading this right now. God gave you a spirit of love, power, and self-discipline, not of fear or timidity! You will regain control of your body! You will regain control of your thoughts and attitude! You will regain control of your emotions in Jesus' name. Your stress does not define you. Only God defines you. So get up, stand tall, and do what it is you need to do to be healthy. I and many others are here for you! All you have to do is ASK!

YOU ARE WORTH IT!

For Reflection:

What are some creative pursuits you engage that help you relax? What are some creative outlets you would like to pursue?

_____

_____

Name three things that you can take control of in your life to stir your passions and seize the day! Share them with someone and commit to make changes.

_____

_____

THE PROCESS OF CHANGE

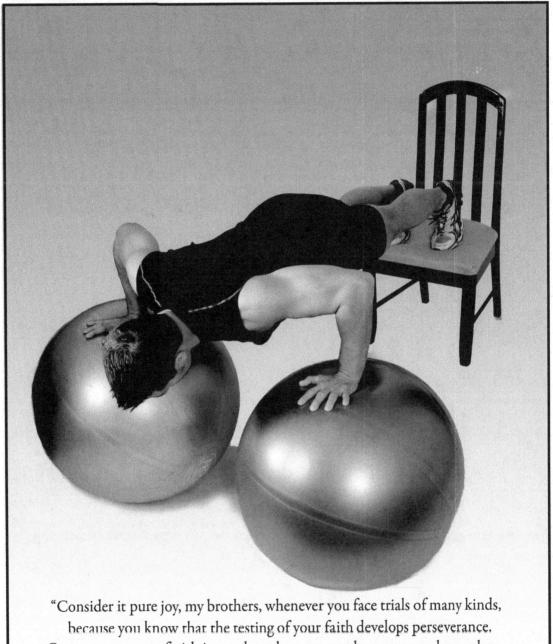

"Consider it pure joy, my brothers, whenever you face trials of many kinds,
because you know that the testing of your faith develops perseverance.
Perseverance must finish its work so that you may be mature and complete,
not lacking anything." (James 1:2)

WEEK SIX

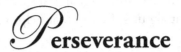

Perseverance

"The process of change"

By now, for many of you the honeymoon is over. It's week 6 and the initial motivation and excitement you once had with your exercise and nutrition has probably worn off. Why? Why is change so hard when it comes to creating a healthy lifestyle? Imagine a mountain for a moment. What needs to happen for you to reach the summit? You must *climb* the mountain, right! In essence, without a challenge or battle there is no victory. That sounds fine and dandy, but, I, like many of you have climbed a mountain before and ¾ of the way up, as my lungs and legs were burning like fire from lack of oxygen, I thought, "What have I gotten myself into." This may or may not be where you are. You may be tellng yourself, "This mountain is just too big!" Well, tighten your boots and take a drink of water because you are about to learn how to reach the summit!

It's called perseverence! You have learned how to identify and change your behavior through the "I Am" declaration and the TAP principle. But this doesn't happen only once. It is a process that must be repeated every day. Perseverance is the time and energy it takes to continue in the process to reach the peak. Perseverance is a journey and serves a very important function in your life. It is crucial in your spiritual maturity and the strengthening of your faith.

> **"Consider it pure joy, my brothers, when you face trials of many kinds, because you know that the testing of your faith develops perseverance. Perseverance must finish its work so that you may be mature and complete, not lacking anything."** (James 1:2–4)

Does this mean waiting on the trials of life to humble you? No! To learn the concept of perseverance, you need activities that specifically build and strengthen your persevering nature. In other words, don't just wait for life to cause you to persevere—go out of your way to create things in your life that *require* you to persevere. **Physical exercise is a fundamental tool to help you become spiritually mature because of the perseverance needed to become and stay healthy.**

God designed you with the capacity to overcome adversity. Remember, like Jesus, you are called to take action, and every action has a process or time-frame. **The process of this action over time is perseverance and produces life-change.** Perseverance is beautiful because it reveals the Christ-like warrior in you.

Perseverance always involves some degree of human suffering, which is possibly the reason that so many of you don't like to exercise and why many of you have thought of quitting. But if you truly know, or want to know, Jesus Christ, how can you not embrace the beautiful reality of suffering and its importance in your life? **The physiological experience of perseverance is**

suffering. True love sometimes means suffering, as Jesus ultimately showed us on His journey to the cross. But what exactly is it about suffering that helps you and nurtures you? The answer is found in Romans:

> **We also rejoice in our sufferings, because we know that suffering produces perseverance; perseverance, character; and character, hope. And hope does not disappoint us, because God has poured out his love into our hearts by the Holy Spirit, whom he has given us."** (Romans 5:3–5)

Does this scripture make reference only to emotional or spiritual suffering? No. Suffering is suffering. This means any form of suffering produces the same results of perseverance, character, and then hope. God is so amazing that He even created you to benefit from any kind of suffering. Suffering is never in vain!

All of this means that if you willingly and purposefully take yourself through a temporary form of physical suffering by exercising, you will be strengthened. God also demonstrates this principle when He tells you to fast and pray. When you fast and pray, you humble yourself and suffer before God. In this willful and purposeful display of temporary suffering, you are strengthened by God because the results in Romans 5:3–5 apply to *every* type of suffering. God is faithful and holds true to His word and promises 100% of the time. In essence, physical exercise and fasting are integral to your spiritual maturity. **Willingly and purposefully taking yourself through a temporary form of physical suffering via exercise enables you to better handle those times and events in life that are beyond your control—when suffering is not voluntary. It is a way to help prepare you in advance for the trials of life.**

So why has it been so difficult to discipline yourself to exercise and eat right? The answer is that you have been living each day with the same patterns or behaviors, and when you step out of those patterns or behaviors, even though they are bad ones, it is painful. Change isn't easy. God makes you look deep into your life, and sometimes you won't like what He shows you. The key to change is finding the courage and godly motivation to change and then to persevere when your natural tendency is to give up.

There is always a price to pay during the journey or process of undergoing positive life-change of any kind, and God will make *you* make the changes so *you* can overcome them. Perseverance is the time it takes for this change to happen. And in this process of perseverance, you will find out if the goal of your faith is genuine or not.

> **". . . though now for a little while you may have had to suffer grief in all kinds of trials. These have come so that your faith—of greater worth than gold, which perishes even though refined by fire—may be proved genuine and may result in praise, glory, and honor when Jesus Christ is revealed."** (1 Peter 1:6–7)

This even applies to you as you begin an exercise and eating program. It doesn't just mean when you surrender your life to Christ for the first time. You are supposed to surrender to Christ *daily!* Many of you have never surrendered your health to Christ, and it is time you did! Christ will test you to see if the goal or commitment you have made to better your health is genuine or not. *It isn't supposed to be easy.*

Our society looks at the words *perseverance* and *suffering* as negative. They usually remind us of something we have gone through that is difficult. We associate perseverance and suffering with pain and hardship. After all, that is what suffering is, right?

4 Profiles in Perseverance

Profile 1

During a seminar on perseverance I gave at a north Houston YMCA, we came to the question in the *Courage to Change Life Application Journal* that states: "Name an area in your life where you have had to persevere through something physical." What followed was amazing. A woman in the class looked somber as she reluctantly yet confidently shared that she had to overcome cancer five years earlier. With tears rolling down her face, she shared the many hardships she had faced and the perseverance she had needed to survive. She talked about how different her life was and how many changes she had to make as a result of having cancer.

During the first six weeks of her training and seminars, she struggled with her nutrition. It was hard for her to make the changes she needed to make. She was frustrated because her faith in God was strong, and she was a very spiritually-mature Christian woman, yet she just couldn't seem to get a handle on things. As we talked about her battle with cancer and the struggles she had persevered through, however, I realized that the root of her frustration was the root that so many of us share in our battle with making better choices with our fitness and nutrition.

Because of her cancer, she associated perseverance with pain and sickness. So as she went through the program and was called on to physically persevere through the exercise and nutrition changes, the feelings of perseverance were familiarly negative and recalled her life-threatening battle with cancer.

Profile 2

Another woman in the class had lost her son years ago, and some of the perseverance she needed to be successful during the program was associated with (or attached to) the emotional pain of losing her son. She had not realized that she was carrying that "weight" around. Once she did realize it, she dealt with it head-on! Remember that *suffering is the physiological experience of perseverance.* It is actually a physical experience, even though what happened may have been emotional. Oftentimes, it is physical *and* emotional, as with the woman who had cancer. So unless we have a paradigm shift in how we view perseverance and suffering, we will always associate them with pain and trauma.

Who wants to start an exercise program if the subconscious feelings of pain, hurt, and sickness will surface during the process of persevering? All of us have been through things that were hard, life-threatening, and just plain bad. So it is no wonder why it is so difficult to persevere through positive life-changes while making healthy choices! My goodness!

Profile 3

Another woman in the same class had suffered through a very bad and abusive marriage. She shared with us the story of how she had finally left her abusive husband even as he was holding her at gunpoint. In time she had healed, but the physical feeling of perseverance was still connected to pain and trauma. She was reminded not only of the perseverance she had needed after leaving the abusive marriage, but she also had to deal with her guilt and shame for persevering through something she probably should not have—putting up with many years of physical and mental abuse when God had wanted her safe and out of harm's way. At the six-week mark of the *Courage to Change* program she, too, was having trouble sticking to (or persevering through) her commitment to better her health. During the seminar, she openly forgave herself, and the one who had abused her, and was further set free from guilt and shame. She and the others began to open themselves to the beauty and positive power of perseverance.

Profile 4

My final story is that of a precious client and friend I have trained for quite some time. She is one of those dream clients who makes me laugh as we train. We have a great time. She began training with me two years after becoming a widow. We talked often about her husband and the wonderful life they had shared together. Tears usually flowed as we took that trip down memory lane.

One day I asked her if she was doing well on her nutrition. She confessed that she was struggling a little, especially with the feeling of hunger. She told me it always felt as if she were depriving herself when she felt hungry. We talked about the importance of feeling the hunger and how it related to staying tapped into God—as a form of fasting. Though it wasn't fasting in the sense of not eating, it was in the sense of feeling the body ask for food after the high-octane food wears off and is burned up. Feeling this hunger is actually healthy because it is a reminder that our bodies need nourishment to live and flourish. That was all fine and dandy and she understood all of it, but the root was waiting for both of us.

Here was where the breakthrough came. I asked her to think back over the past two years and remember how she felt as she was missing her husband. I asked her specifically to remember what her physical body felt like. Tears began to flow as I helped her put the puzzle pieces in place. **The physical feeling of the loss of her husband was almost identical to the feeling of physical hunger she experienced as she made healthy choices. It was such a familiar feeling that it sabotaged her ability to stay on a good nutrition plan.**

She didn't realize that by persevering through the familiar feelings, she was actually opening herself up to further healing from the loss of her husband and further healing in her body. See, there is a chemical bond or connection that happens to married couples as they share their lives together. As they sleep next to each other every night as well as make love, their bodies become chemically interlaced. As she grieved for her husband emotionally, a physical grieving also had to take place. Her body missed that chemical bond and connection she had shared with her husband. Realizing this was a major breakthrough for her. She left the training session with renewed strength and optimism. She knew it would not be easy to persevere through some of those familiar feelings of loss as she felt hungry, but, she understood the root of her struggles and how the perseverance related to healing both her body and her grief. What a powerful lesson!

The dangerous pleasure of chemical dependency

That same principle of chemical dependency in our marital relationships is found in food itself. Though many factors are in play, there is actually a chemical dependency or addiction in a culture centered on food. Houston, Texas, is an example of a city whose entire culture is centered on food. This is what actually happens in food dependency or addiction. A chemical—the pleasure hormone dopamine (from which our word "dope" derives)—gets released in the brain when we engage in a pleasurable activity such as eating. Dopamine gives us a feeling of well-being and pleasure. Without exercise, we have to eat more and more and more to get the same effect of dopamine, similar to developing a tolerance to a drug we become addicted to. As we literally feed the addiction, it takes more and more food to give us the high (of pleasure) we are seeking. The interesting thing is that exercise releases the same hormone (dopamine) as making love with your spouse. But which is easier and more fun—eating more or exercising? Ooh, I just heard some sighs.

Let's say a woman decreases her calorie intake without exercising. Her body goes into a withdrawal because dopamine is not giving her the "high" that she is addicted to. It is a vicious cycle. The lower level of dopamine gives you a feeling of deprivation very similar to the feeling my client experienced when she lost her husband. Some people gain a lot of weight after losing a spouse because they crave the "high" from dopamine as they overeat. It acts as a surrogate "fix" for the chemicals the body is missing from the person who passed away. Only exercise can safely satisfy the body's need for dopamine. Weight training and cardiovascular exercise are crucially important. It is a divine design—a way for God to keep us active, physically and emotionally healed, and on top of our game. He wants us to always be in an action mindset full of strength, endurance, stamina, and energy, all of which take a lot of perseverance to be successful. Thus we can truly be free within ourselves and have the energy to serve others effectively!

Life Happens!

We have had to persevere through adversity during the process of publishing this book. In the two years prior to the book's publication my wife and I were in two car accidents that occurred because someone wasn't paying attention and crashed into us. The first accident sent Silesia to the hospital with back injuries, and she has suffered two years of back pain. I pulled all the muscles in the left side of my neck, which drastically hampered my ability to workout and do everyday activities as I like to. Three months after the second accident, a woman driving in front of me panicked while crossing a railroad track. When the lights began blinking she decided (at the last moment) that she couldn't make it in time, so she slammed on her breaks, threw her car into reverse, and slammed into me. More neck therapy.

During that same time period, we had a chronically ill child whom we had to homebound school for two years. After a year we saw a specialist and found out that he had been misdiagnosed. The specialist discovered that our son did not have enough antibodies to fight off infection. He was given a shot to boost his antibodies and it worked. However, during the year-long timeframe of misdiagnosis, though, he had been put on high doses of antibiotics and steroids—over and over and over—which only caused him to become sicker. So another year of misdiagnosis passed until we found out that his body had an illness called Candida, a build up of nasty fungus in his body that was a direct result of overusing antibiotics. After a lot of prayer we finally found the solution and just as we got him back to 100%, and as he was looking forward to school, football, and getting out of the house with friends again, he fell off his bike while going pretty fast, fractured his skull, and suffered a double concussion. He had internal bleeding, the works. He is OK now. Thank you God!

As if all that weren't enough, seven weeks prior to the photo shoot for this book I broke my ribs while water skiing. To make things worse, I felt horrible physically for well over a year. I had no energy, no drive, and was exhausted all the time. My muscle mass went down and my body fat went up. My feet hurt, hands hurt, body ached, and would take an entire week to recover from one simple workout. I thought it was merely stress. Just before I turned 40, though, my wife was listening to a doctor on the radio talk about the symptoms in men who suffer from low testosterone. Through her intervention and encouragement I got myself checked out. My doctor discovered and confirmed that my hormone (testosterone) levels were dangerously low and she started me on therapy. While my energy was slowly coming back, Silesia also had to go for therapy for a torn meniscus in her knee. Oh, and did I mention we also went through two major hurricanes—Rita and Ike—in this same timeframe? We had major wind and water damage and no electricity for which seemed to be an eternity. The final 5 weeks of editing this book, before sending everything in to the publisher, Silesia came down with a strange virus. What was frustrating was that Silesia was doing everything right regarding exercise and nutrition before she got sick. Even as I write this now it has lasted 5 weeks and the doctors are telling us to wait it out. And let's not talk about the fact that during those 5 weeks all three cars broke down costing us over 4 grand.

Friends, life happens and sometimes it seems to never end. Believe me when I say, "We understand!" But we push on. We CAN NOT and WILL NOT let the adversity we persevere through cause us to lose site of being healthy and joyful; or to quit! Not only was it difficult to continue working out and taking care of ourselves as a family in the midst of all that turmoil, but it was also very difficult to literally persevere through the *Courage to Change*, to build the very book and program you are reading now. Silesia and I still had to stay connected, exercise and eat right as best we could, minister to and take care of our family, make a living, run our business, and run a household. The books came after all of that. But as a family we pushed through. We persevered and are continuing to persevere. There is value to everything we went through and everything we will go through. And there is value in your hardships, too, if you will lean on God's very big shoulders.

Can you see how easy it is for all of us to associate negativity and pain with what we have to persevere through, even if it is something (such as good nutrition and exercise) that is good for us? Can you see why so many of us have had trouble persevering through a commitment we have made? Can you see how important it is to change your view of perseverance and suffering from a negative to a positive? Can you see how willingly and purposefully taking yourself through a temporary form of physical suffering via exercise enables you to better handle those times and events in life that are beyond your control? Can you see how persevering in your commitment to your health is a huge part of your spiritual maturity? Can you see now why God says to "rejoice in our sufferings, because we know that suffering produces perseverance, character, and hope. And hope does not disappoint us, because God has poured out His love into our hearts by the Holy Spirit, whom He has given us" (Romans 5:3–5)?

Give God whatever pain and hardships you have associated with perseverance. Do this so you can embrace perseverance as a powerful positive force in your life and not a negative one. The perseverance you need to fulfill your health goals, wedding vows, parental responsibilities, and job duties depends on your ability to experience perseverance as beautiful, energizing, and empowering!

Persevere, pay the price, and gain the victory of good health inside and out!

For Reflection:

Share a time in your life when you have persevered and what positive effects you experienced as a result.

_____

_____

Share a time in your life when you have not persevered and what negative effects you experienced as a result.

_____

_____

Can you identify any pain that you associate with perseverance?

_____

_____

The Pain of Love

"The art of intercession"

Have you ever noticed the physical pain you feel while supporting someone? How do you feel when you are with a friend or relative who is hurting? Think of the physical pain you feel when someone you love dies or when your children are messing up in school or rebelling against you. What exactly is this pain? Where does it come from? The answer is beautiful.

As you let Christ live in your heart and lead you in your daily life, Christ in you will use you to intercede for others. **"Christ Jesus, who died—more than that, who was raised to life—is at the right hand of God and is also interceding for us"** (Romans 8:34). And since Jesus also says in John 14:20, **"I am in my Father, and you are in me, and I am in you,"** you will begin to see how God uses you to intercede for those around you. You are a part of Jesus and Jesus is a part of you. In this love affair between you and Christ, you will share in and physically feel the **"pain of love"** on behalf of those for whom you are interceding.

Your spirit seeks and craves the deep things of God, and it is in your spirit that you intercede for others. The Holy Spirit ministers to your spirit and puts people on your heart to pray for. **"In the same way, the Spirit helps us in our weakness. We do not know what we ought to pray for, but the Spirit himself intercedes for us with groans that words cannot express. And he who searches our hearts knows the mind of the Spirit, because the Spirit intercedes for the saints in accordance with God's will"** (Romans 8:26–27). Because our bodies house our spirits and are home to the Holy Spirit, intercession is manifested in our physical bodies. That is why we "feel" the heaviness as we intercede for people. This shows all of us that we are here to build loving intimate relationships. (We will consider this in detail in Week 10.)

So why have I included a section on intercession in a book about health and fitness? Because no matter how God asks you to intercede for others, a physical response and a heaviness come with it. You *physically* feel the pain and stress from those for whom you intercede. I call it the **"pain of love."** In Matthew 11:29–30, Jesus tells us, **"Take my yoke upon you and learn from me, for I am gentle and humble in heart, and you will find rest for your souls. For my yoke is easy and my burden is light."**

"My burden is light" is what sticks out. Jesus does not tell us that there will be **no** burden or that we will never experience pain. There *is* a burden as we follow Jesus, and your physical body will always feel this. Think back to a time when you have been worried about someone you love and care for and recall how your body felt. It felt heavy, didn't it?

Oftentimes as you intercede for someone, the physical burden you experience will feel as though it is more than you can bear. Is it more than you can bear because God has given you too much, or is it possibly because your body is so out of shape that any extra stress or heaviness causes an overload? Think hard about that. Your body will always share the experience of what you are going through spiritually! It can be either an aid or a hindrance to you. How well you take care of yourself will dictate which it is.

Unless you keep your body strong and healthy, you will not have the strength to serve as God asks you. The stronger you are and the more physical endurance you gain, the better able you are to intercede for others so that you can help them heal and grow by your sharing in their pain and suffering. Physical exercise is a beautiful way to give that pain of love you took from them back to God. After all, Jesus is the greatest of all intercessors. He not only died on the cross to intercede for our sins but His spirit intercedes for us daily to help us grow and heal from the things we go through.

This is a powerful lesson that we all need to learn. When done correctly and for the right reasons or motives, nutrition and exercise are not vain activities. Rather, they are a beautiful way for us to stay connected to each other and stay strong as we share in each other's physical "pains of love" and bear one another's burdens (Galatians 6:2).

For Reflection:

Have you ever experienced the "pain of love" in your own life? When?

_____

_____

What does Brian mean when he says that healthy nutrition and exercise are not vain pursuits? Can you make this connection to your own life? Explain.

_____

_____

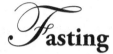asting

"Both physical and spiritual cleansing"

Fasting, like physical exercise, is a fundamental tool to help you become spiritually mature because you need perseverance to go through with it. As with physical exercise, in fasting you willingly and purposefully take yourself through a temporary form of physical suffering. This enables you to better handle those times and events in life that are beyond your control. Fasting helps prepare you in advance for the trials of life.

Fasting is a lost art that needs to be revived. Many—I would say *most*—Christians have never actually fasted. That is a shame because the rewards are beautiful. Let us revive this wonderful tool of physical and spiritual cleansing.

What happens when you abstain from eating? You begin to die. Your body craves nourishment and calories to survive. When you deny your body this basic need, you must rely on strength from God to fill you up. This teaches you what Jesus said in Matthew 4:4, **"Jesus answered, 'It is written: Man does not live on bread alone, but on every word that comes from the mouth of God.'"**

Fasting provides not only a spiritual cleansing but a physical cleansing as well. They again happen simultaneously. As you fast and pray, you will gain self-control on all levels, including the importance of eating healthy food once you begin eating again.

Oftentimes, we do not truly appreciate something until it is gone. Do you live to eat or do you eat to live? As you fast you will answer this question. As your body begins to weaken, you will learn that you eat to live by providing your body with good, nutritious food. Does this mean that you are never going to have a cheeseburger or pizza again? No! It means that you will make better, more responsible decisions as you take care of yourself. Many of us do not even get hungry because our metabolism is so out of whack. As you fast, you will begin to feel those hunger pangs telling you that your body is missing something and that it is time to refuel. As we saw in many of the stories I have shared, this will also help many of you heal as your body's perception of what perseverance is changes. That feeling of hunger will change from a bad memory to a reminder of the suffering that Jesus went through on the cross. This reminder should not make you feel bad, it should empower you to further live in freedom and joy!

As you deny your body this need for food and God gives you the strength, you will gain the self-control you need to avoid all the temptations and cravings once you are able to eat again. As you fast, I recommend that you keep it between yourself and God.

"**When you fast, do not look somber as the hypocrites do, for they disfigure their faces to show men they are fasting. I tell you the truth, they have received their reward in full. But when you fast, put oil on your head and wash your face, so that it will not be obvious to men that you are fasting, but only to your Father, who is unseen; and your Father, who sees what is done in secret, will reward you.**" (Matthew 6:16–18)

If you do it out of boastfulness and pride, the benefits will not be there. You will just be very hungry and all you will think about is eating again. **Fasting with the right motives will give you spiritual insight into your life, strength, a renewed vision and purpose, and a stronger connection to God.**

Fasting with your husband, wife, colleagues, and friends can also be beneficial. Sharing in the fasting experience is a way to bring all of you closer together, to further support and encourage each other as you all take back authority in your lives. Watch as you grow together, enhance the intimacy between you, and build an even stronger foundation on God for your relationships. Entire offices, Bible study groups, and families can participate in a fast together. Again, be silent and do not boast or outwardly talk about what you are doing with people unless they specifically ask. Once it is over, come together as a group and discuss your experience. Your *Life Application Journal* will help you with this.

Two Types of Fasting

So how long should you fast? Let's start by defining two types of fasting. The first type of fasting is *out of sacrifice*, and the second is *out of obedience*. When you decide to fast by your own desire because you want to cleanse yourself, it is out of self-sacrifice—you are willingly denying yourself food to become spiritually stronger and physically disciplined. This is a good thing. But sometimes the Holy Spirit will specifically put on your heart to fast for and intercede for someone, or for some event, you need to be spiritually strong for. As you listen and do what has been put on your heart, you are fasting out of obedience. It takes a while to become spiritually developed enough to listen this closely, but the rewards are amazing. And even the most mature Christian doesn't always get it right!

Many mornings I have awakened and felt the need to fast. Later in the day I would learn why. Before Silesia and I came together, I waited for her for about three years. She had gone through a very long struggle, and I knew that it was just too painful for her to love again. I felt the Holy Spirit telling me to wait for her to heal from the wounds of her painful past. While waiting for Silesia, there were periods of four to six months when I would have no contact with her at all—no telephone, e-mail, nothing. Even though I would have no contact with her, I would periodically feel the pain of something she was going through. One morning I woke up at 4:00 a.m. with a horrible stomachache. The funny thing was that I woke up actually praying for her in my sleep, out loud. I knew that what I was feeling was not from me but from *her*. The Holy Spirit had me intercede for her, to share some of the burden of something painful she was going through. So I prayed and prayed for her all morning, fasted the rest of the day, and journaled that night. About a week after this happened, I found the courage to call her and see if she was all right. We had not spoken in at least four months. I asked her what had been going on with her about 4:00 in the morning a week earlier. She listened in silence as I told her of the physical pain I had felt in my stomach as the Holy Spirit prompted me to pray for her all morning and the rest of the day.

She then proceeded to tell me that she had been in the hospital with stomach and bladder pain and that at that very time when I was interceding she had been in a lot of pain. Though at the time it kind of freaked her out, she knew in her spirit that God had used me to intercede for her and to share with her the **"pain of love." Silesia has been used by God numerous times to fast and pray for me too. In fact, it amazes me the amount of people, close and distant, she lovingly and willingly intercedes for all the time.** Fasting has become a huge part of our life. I encourage all of you to embrace this long lost art. Again, your *Life Application Journal* will help you do this.

When starting to fast by your own desire, I would recommend starting after dinner one night. Go through the entire next day without eating and end your fast the following morning with a wonderful healthy breakfast—*not* a slab of bacon cooked in lard. Make sure that you drink as much water as you can while fasting. Chewing sugar-free, calorie-free gum is also a good idea because fasting can cause bad breath. Not eating takes your body into ketosis, where your body goes to your protein for energy. If you are fasting out of obedience to the Holy Spirit, stay in tune because the Holy Spirit will also tell you when it is over. Do the best you can. You aren't always going to do it perfectly. Know how much God loves you and that He is there to help you be as strong as you can be at all times.

And as always, **consult your physician before fasting. Fasting isn't for everyone. Some of you have diabetes, hypoglycemia, and other ailments that make fasting a very bad idea.** This is another reason you need to be healthy. You need to be healthy enough to fast. Otherwise you won't reap the physical *or* spiritual benefits of fasting. So get the OK from your doctor first. Have fun with this and watch as your self-control becomes much stronger.

For Reflection:

If you have ever fasted, describe the experience—physically, mentally, spiritually?

_____

_____

THE CHILD IN YOU

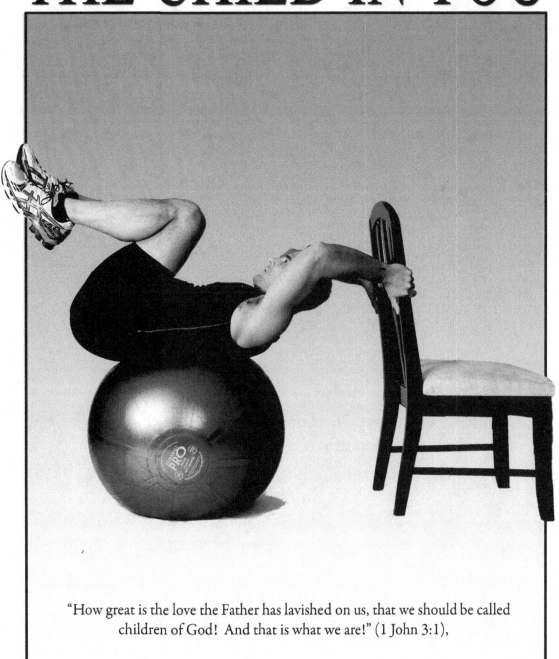

"How great is the love the Father has lavished on us, that we should be called children of God! And that is what we are!" (1 John 3:1),

WEEK SEVEN

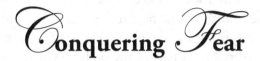

Conquering Fear

"Reclaiming, owning, and living the promises of God"

Let's begin Week 7 with a look at the life of a *Courage to Change* participant named Ruth. Her greatest breakthroughs came as she conquered fear and took ownership of who she was and stepped into her true birthright, an inheritance of love and power. What had happened to cause her to *not* live this way for most of her life? Ruth's early life was difficult. In fact, it was horrific. As a young child she saw her father gunned down on the front porch of their home in a drive-by shooting. After witnessing her father's death, her uncle came to live with the family. Her life went from bad to worse. For the rest of her youth her uncle molested her daily. She lived in constant fear. Until recently Ruth treated herself the way she had been treated, just as so many of you do. We associate our worth with how others treat us and then treat ourselves the same way. See, Ruth struggled with her weight most of her life. Because of her past, she was crippled emotionally and spiritually. She felt ugly and didn't feel worthy of being pretty. In some ways she wanted herself to be invisible to men, unattractive and not desirable. Years of sexual abuse stole from her the right to feel sexy, attractive, and desirable. The acts that caused this were physical, yes, but the only way she could take back control of her physical body was through spiritual healing and restoration.

Her only experience with a father and a father-figure was murder and molestation, so she had to learn who her true Father was and what His intentions were for her. She had to learn that her circumstances were outside of her. This is very difficult for a woman who has been raped or molested. She had to learn to replace the overwhelming fear she had lived in for so long with God's promises and believe in her heart, mind, and soul that she was worthy of receiving them. She had to learn that she did not exercise and take care of herself to make herself more valuable or more beautiful, but rather because she *is* valuable and *is* beautiful! As she did the spiritual work, she also did the physical work. She came to her *Courage to Change* personal training classes twice per week at Grace Community Church in Clear Lake, Texas, and pushed through her fear as she **took her body back!** She deserved to feel sexy, desirable, and beautiful. Because she started "believing" that she was worthy of these feelings, her actions supported her belief through the changes she made for her health. She changed her nutrition habits, exercise habits, thought habits, everything! She conquered her fear by reclaiming, owning, and living the promises of God which were then made manifest in how she treated herself! *Go Ruth!*

The Only Thing to Fear...

As you can see, one of the greatest obstacles you face as you move forward with *Courage to Change* is fear. In your spiritual heritage you will find the will to take care of yourself and the ability to conquer fear. Any fear or oppression that you allow in your life, either knowingly or unknowingly, will keep you from walking in your heritage. Even if you love Jesus Christ with all of your heart, the enemy is sneaky and will find ways of keeping you from your heritage. Fear is the greatest of these poisons. It is time to reclaim the heritage the Lord has promised you, to walk in His confidence and power in everything you do. God set your heritage before you were born. Think of your heritage as your birthright. As part of the body of Christ, you are a member of a royal family who deserves all the royal treatment and privileges. It is time you started acting like it. Isaiah 54:13–17 tells us how to conquer fear:

> **"All your sons will be taught by the LORD, and great will be your children's peace. In righteousness you will be established. Tyranny will be far from you. You will have nothing to fear. Terror will be far removed; it will not come near you. If anyone does attack you, it will not be my doing; whoever attacks you will surrender to you. See, it is I who created the blacksmith who fans the coals into flame and forges a weapon fit for its work. And it is I who have created the destroyer to work havoc. No weapon forged against you will prevail, and you will refute every tongue that accuses you. This is the heritage of the servants of the LORD, and this is their vindication from me, declares the LORD."**

The heritage God speaks of here makes no reference to your health because your heritage is not an action from you. Rather, it is a promise and action from God. But, reclaiming or recapturing your heritage *is* the result of *your* actions, how you follow Jesus and live your life each moment with love. All of the promises of God deal directly with overcoming fear.

Promise #1: "All your sons (and daughters) will be taught by the LORD"

God is faithful. God always fulfills His promises. Not 88% of the time, not 98% of the time, but 100% of the time! Church services, Bible studies, classes, pastors, mentors, friends, and family can all help build your relationship with Jesus, but God himself promises to personally teach you as well! Much of what we fear comes from what we do not know, and God's promise is to teach us. It is up to you to listen and obey. He loves you just as much as He loves every other person in the world and wants you to walk every day in the victory of your heritage. Take ownership of His promise to teach you and replace the fear with courage and confidence that God is with you. He will teach you courage, give you wisdom to take care of yourself, and teach you discipline regarding your health, relationships, and career. He will teach you thankfulness for your body and the ability to take care of yourself with exercise and good nutrition. And He will teach you how to be faithful to Him in your commitments regarding your health and life in general.

This promise, as well as all of the others you will soon learn, is twofold and comes with a powerful legacy. God promises to teach not only *you* as His child but your children as well. Part of your heritage is a powerful legacy to your children and your children's children. As you raise them up in the Lord and pass on His legacy to them, God promises to personally teach them as well. **Your children learn from you through your actions, and they learn from God through their actions.** (Read that again!) Sure, they learn to own positive words, scripture, and encouragement as you speak truth into and over their lives, but it is in your *actions* of love and authority that they learn to claim their inheritance and be free from fear. What behavior would you have your children learn from you—good, healthy living, or destructive lifestyle choices dictated by fear? **Their ability to hear from and be personally taught by the Lord as part of their heritage, or birthright, depends largely on your ability to pass on the legacy of God with your healthy actions leading the way.**

Promise #2: "And great will be your children's peace"

As you let Him teach you courage for a healthier lifestyle and your actions reinforce that courage, God promises to give you peace. Fear robs you of peace and joy and paralyzes you. True peace transcends every area of your life as you look to Jesus and honor Him with your actions and obedience. But He doesn't just say *a little peace*, or that once in a while, He will give you peace. He says **"GREAT will be your children's peace."** You deserve to walk in the freedom and peace of a lean, healthy body with a sound mind and confident emotions, not in timidity, self-doubt, and self-destructive behavior. Why? Because it is your heritage to do so, and it is a promise that God will fulfill 100% of the time as you follow Him.

How many of you feel shame, guilt, and/or fear regarding your health? How many of you battle with insecurities, doubt, and condemning thoughts regarding your weight and body image? Remember that how you overcome these things and reclaim your heritage is what passes the legacy of peace onto your children. Sure, they sometimes stray, but once they have the foundation of God built in them, which you provided by your actions, they usually find their way back into His arms. "And great will be your children's peace." Let His promise to give you and your children peace be enough for you to carry on and conquer your fear.

Promise #3: "In righteousness you will be established"

Oh my goodness, this one is worthy of an entire book in itself because it is through Jesus Christ that you are established. This is a promise from God that when you welcome Jesus into your heart, the blood of Jesus will sustain you through all things. Does fear establish you, or define you, or does Jesus? Does your obedience, or disobedience, establish you, or does Jesus? Only Jesus Christ can establish you. This entire book has been written to show you that.

Promise #4: "Tyranny will be far from you"

Recall how I said earlier that the biggest reason for poor health is not a lack of exercise or nutrition programs, health clubs, or even good personal trainers, but the spiritual oppression or tyranny present in your life. Oppression is basically an attack of the enemy designed to keep you from walking in your heritage. Oppression shows up in many different forms, such as fear, confusion, complacency, condemnation, insecurities, unworthiness, and pride. These are just a few of the ways you become spiritually oppressed. They affect your will to take care of yourself. Think of oppression or tyranny as bondage, something holding you down and paralyzing you from doing the action you need to accomplish your dreams and goals, operating in the healthy will of God.

As you go to God and follow Him in all you do, He promises to keep oppression or tyranny far from you. He doesn't just say "away from you," He says "*far from you.*" There *is* hope in the promises of God, and you *will* learn to take back your birthright, a life free from tyranny and oppression. You will then live in the freedom of a good, healthy lifestyle.

Some forms of oppression are passed down from generation to generation in families, and some we take on by our own disobedience and unhealthy lifestyles. When you overcome the source of this oppression by the power of Jesus Christ, you will walk in the heritage God has promised you. The greatest lesson about tyranny is that it is *outside* of you. Tyranny comes when you take something that has happened and own it by taking it inside of you and letting it affect and control you. Jesus said, **"I am in the father and the father is in me and I am in you!"** Nothing in this world can enter you if you truly know *who* is in you. A major objective of this book is to teach you how to identify what is in you that is keeping you from your heritage and to empower you to take out the trash so you can live free from the oppression or tyranny inside you. Another book I recommend that deals with oppression in detail is *Shadow Boxing* by Dr. Henry Malone. Always be on the lookout for books and classes—perhaps hosted in your own church—that help you overcome spiritual oppression. Get involved! My *"Faith in Action"* seminars based on this book and the *Life Application Journal* also help you fight back and equip you with powerful tools to reclaim your heritage by taking back the authority in your life.

Promise #5: "You will have nothing to fear. Terror will be far removed; it will not come near you"

This promise is one of the most important. How many of you live in fear of some kind? How many of you feel paralyzed to act regarding your health? How many of you are sick and tired of being afraid of rejection, ridicule, and laughter regarding your health? How many of you are insecure with your own spouse and are afraid of how you look to him or her? Many of you will not even let yourselves acknowledge the fear in your lives because it has taken such a deep root in you. As I discussed earlier, God is here right now, waiting to show you how to overcome fear and live each moment in the beautiful present. His promise to you is that you will have nothing to fear. Terror will be far removed and it will not come near you. The fact that God says "it" will not come near you means that fear is a force, or actual spirit, and not just a state of mind. Fear or terror is a manifestation of the enemy trying to keep you from claiming and walking in your heritage. The spirit of fear will always exist because we live in a fallen world. God promises that as you take back your authority, "Terror will be far removed; it will not come near you." And you wonder why it has been so hard to take care of yourself, to stand firm in your healthy commitments!

The reason God promises that you will have nothing to fear is because He designed you to overcome fear. Why did God tell Joshua to **"Be strong and courageous, do not be afraid or discouraged, for the Lord God is with you wherever you go"** (Joshua 1:9)? He said this to Joshua over and over because he was afraid, that's why! God is the ultimate encourager, and with His strength and courage you can push forward and conquer any fear just as Joshua did, no matter how hard your task may seem. There is only one thing you are to fear—God. Deuteronomy 5:29 says, **"Oh, that their hearts would be inclined to fear me and keep all my commands always, so that it might go well with them and their children forever!"**

Bottom line: What you fear, you manifest! So, what do you fear? If you fear that your relationship with your husband or wife will end in divorce, it probably will because you then manifest it with your actions, even without knowing it. If you fear that you will never get a job promotion or that you will never be happy in your career, you probably won't because your behavior manifests it. Even vowing that you will never act like your abusive parents did will make it likely that you will manifest those same undesirable qualities because your vow was made out of fear instead of out of your allegiance to Christ.

If you vow to lose weight out of fear, you will eventually go right back to where you were even if you do lose it for a while because the vow was made from fear. How many times have you been through this "yo-yo syndrome"? If you fear losing weight, you may never lose weight because your body simply responds to what you believe in with faith and the actions that follow. **In essence you are putting your faith in fear instead of placing your faith in the power of the Lord.**

Deuteronomy 5:29 is so powerful because it is showing you that as you fear the Lord it will "go well with them and their children forever!" How well you deal with fear not only helps you reclaim your heritage, but leaves a powerful legacy to your children. Why are some diseases generational? Why do heart disease, cancer, diabetes, and other diseases sometimes "run in families" (i.e., show up in a family's blood line)? Many times it is caused by fears of these things that have been passed down from generation to generation, thus manifesting them by the fear and unhealthy actions that follow.

Fear leads to paralysis, paralysis leads to sickness, and sickness leads to death. To fear the world and its circumstances is to manifest the world and its circumstances. All eating disorders are fear based because a control issue from either the past or the future is present. The person is either holding on to some trauma of the past, or is in fear of being fat in the future, sometimes caught in a vicious cycle of both. A thin person who fears getting fat will manifest that mindset and always *feel* fat regardless of how thin he or she is. This is how anorexia and bulimia develop. *What they fear, they manifest.* If you fear that you won't lose weight and will fail at your commitments, you will manifest that failure through your thoughts, attitude, and performance. (Remember the TAP principle.) But you have the power to change that!

What happens if you fear love? Do you manifest it? Absolutely not, because ultimately it isn't love you fear. *It is impossible to fear love.* **"There is no fear in love. But perfect love drives out fear, because fear has to do with punishment. The one who fears is not made perfect in love"** (1 John 4:18). What you fear instead of love is hurt, betrayal, rejection, or maybe abuse. As you fear these things you bring them into your physical reality and even push people away—people who have nothing but pure intentions for your life.

Why does perfect love drive out fear and why are we to fear God? Are you ready for this? The answer is simple and beautiful! *To fear God is to manifest God.*

> **"Only God is pure love, and when it is Him you fear, the old fear is replaced with His qualities, the fruit of His Spirit: love, joy, peace, patience, kindness, goodness, faithfulness, gentleness, and self-control (temperance)."** (Galatians 5:22)

You fear God out of reverence, humility, and His amazing awesomeness, not out of a hellfire-and-brimstone mindset. He created all that is good. He is all-loving, all-knowing, all-inspiring, and all-encouraging. He is all tears, all joy, all beautiful, and the radiance of everything pure and holy. He is pure light, and there is no darkness in Him. As you fear Him, you manifest all of these qualities plus many, many more, including a wonderful desire to take care of yourself.

As God takes your fear away and replaces it with Himself, you will learn to love yourself and others with "action," which is God's most distinguishing quality. You will also get to look into the future with hope, joy, and a knowingness that God in heaven is watching out for you and that you get to bring the future of what you want into the present.

As you learn to take care of yourself, keep a constant check on where your fear is going. Is it in the Lord out of reverence and awe, or in the things in the world that seem scary? As you live a healthy lifestyle, make better choices, become a better father or mother, son or daughter, place your fear in the Lord and watch as you manifest His amazing love and grace in all you do. And watch as He fulfills His promise to you that **"you will have nothing to fear. Terror will be far removed; it will not come near you."**

Promise #6: "If anyone does attack you, it will not be my doing; whoever attacks you will surrender to you."

God is speaking of His authority and protection here. Part of your heritage is a promise from God that He will protect you and keep you safe. When you realize just how protected you are, fear will be a thing of the past! Does this mean that nothing bad will ever happen to you? No. But how you respond to what happens to you is what keeps you safe and untouchable and away from fear. Remember, it isn't what comes into you that makes you unclean, but what comes out of you. Your attacker will surrender to you because you are called to love him or her. Though bad things sometimes happen to good people (you), the oppression or tyranny present in the act of what happened cannot touch you if you are walking closely with the Lord. This is a promise!

How many of you live with a victim mentality or know someone who does? How many of you live with resentment, blame, revenge, and condemning thoughts toward people who have wronged you in some way? **"Do not take revenge, my friends, but leave room for God's wrath, for it is written: 'It is mine to avenge; I will repay,' says the Lord"** (Romans 12:19). *There is a huge difference between being violated and being victimized.* Many women who have battled with eating disorders and body insecurities were at some point violated by some trauma such as rape, molestation, verbal abuse, neglect, or abandonment. Others have been "victimized" by the marketing and entertainment industry and have bought into the lies of what is considered healthy and attractive.

What happened to these people is horrific and a violation not only of their physical selves but of their spirits as well. But though bad and awful things can and do happen, only *you* can make yourself a victim!

Remember God's Promise #4: "Tyranny will be far from you." The enemy uses events and the evil actions of others to get you to live in fear and oppression. If you stay angry and fearful after being violated in some way, the enemy has accomplished his goal. **He couldn't care less about the event. He simply wants to control you for the rest of your life as a result of it.** The oppression doesn't start until you give the enemy permission to control you. You may not always be able to control what happens to you, but you have complete power and authority over the principalities and oppression that come with any event or evil action staged against you! **Imagine going through a healing and natural grieving process from something that has happened without fear! Doesn't that sound amazing?**

Hear this! Own this!

You are told, "If anyone does attack you, it will not be my doing." God doesn't do harm or bad things. That is the work of the enemy just doing his job. The question is, "Are you doing yours?" Are you fighting back? Are you walking in the authority of God or sitting back blaming everyone else for your misfortunes? God designed you to be a fighter, a warrior. The enemy knows that if He can keep you from living a clean, healthy lifestyle, you won't have the energy to fight. You will walk around beaten, battered, abused, and worn out. Sound familiar? You must be healthy to walk in and reclaim your heritage because only then will you have the strength and perseverance to walk in victory.

The enemy must submit to you and do as you say. He is commanded to surrender to you as part of your heritage. But it is up to you to appropriate or take hold of this promise yourself by taking up your sword, putting on the full armor of God (Ephesians 6:14–17), and being the warrior you were designed to be.

Promise #7: "See, it is I who created the blacksmith who fans the coals into flame and forges a weapon fit for its work"

Promise #8: "And it is I who have created the destroyer to work havoc"

Oh my goodness, why would God create a destroyer whose purpose is to work havoc? The answer is powerful and reveals why God gave you the authority you have. Promises #7 and #8 show you that God Himself created an adversary for you to have authority over! Do you need to read that again? That's right, the enemy was created as a pawn to show you your authority. Yes, there is a destroyer who comes to steal, kill, and destroy (John 10:10), but he is constrained by God to submit to you as you call out the name of Jesus. You were created to be a warrior. Your purpose in life is to work the gifts God has given you as a warrior, to be more than a conqueror (Romans 8:37). That does not mean that bad things will not happen (after all, we live in a fallen world), but the spiritual oppression present during those bad things *must* submit to you as you believe in and actively display the power of God. One of the enemy's prime goals is to riddle you with fear. After all, he is just doing his job. Your job, should you choose to accept it, is to tell him what he can do with that fear and where he can.... Anyway, the weapon you use to make this happen is Christ's love in your life, which leads you into Promise #9!

Promise #9: "No weapon forged against you will prevail"

You were just told in Promises #7 and #8 that you have an adversary whose purpose is to destroy. But if you read Promise #9, you will see that "no weapon forged against you will prevail." Again, that does not mean that nothing bad will ever happen, but it does mean that you *do not* need to fear what comes against you. I believe what God says. If He says "no weapon," then I believe no weapon forged against me will prevail. Nothing—*nothing*—can stand against the power of

Christ's love! Remember, the enemy doesn't really care that much about an event. He cares more about the control and fear you live in as a result of the event. Go back and re-read the story in the Knowledge section in Week 2 of *Courage to Change*. My client's sister was murdered. Though this was a very tragic and horrible event in her life, the enemy took control of her with fear. She made herself morbidly obese out of the false hope that no man would ever find her attractive enough to do the same thing to her. As she faced her fear by losing over 100 pounds of fat, she took a stand, began to heal, and reclaimed her authority. She began to step into her inheritance.

Promise #10: "And you will refute every tongue that accuses you"

Not only will no weapon prevail against you, but you will also refute (prove false or disprove) every tongue that accuses you. There will always be people who come against you. There will always be dream-stealers, abusers, manipulators, cheaters, and controllers. But as you let the love and power of Christ lead you, you will have the courage to stand bold in the face of your accusers and refute them. Those of you involved in court cases may not always get the verdict you want, but standing up and being willing and ready to fight for what is right is what keeps you free from the bondage of oppression and fear. Many of you fear what other people think of you. Many of you let other people's words and accusations dictate your confidence and worth because of fear. Right now is the time to take hold of God's promise that you will refute every tongue that accuses you.

Silesia and I have trained many women clients over the years who have reported that people treat them differently once they start getting healthy. We have heard many stories of women losing weight and getting physically and spiritually stronger only to find that they were no longer invited to company luncheons or get-togethers. Even family members are notorious for being this way. Yes, sadly, even some who claim to know Christ. How often have you allowed other people's insecurities and negativity to drag you down or sabotage your commitments to do what is right? Some of you reading this now might need to be the one who is refuted. We all are from time to time. It is time to turn your wishbone into a backbone and stand firm with who you are and then hear your own powerful voice **refute every tongue that accuses you.**

Promise #11: "This is the heritage of the servants of the LORD"

This is God's signature. God is making you a promise that as you serve and love Him, you are in good hands. God is very thorough. He not only gives you promises but is there to remind you again and again that He has an inheritance waiting for all who love and follow Him. He doesn't say that these things *might* be your heritage. He doesn't say that these things are only for a select part of you. He says, "This *is* the heritage of the servants of the Lord."

Promise #12: "And this is their vindication from me, declares the LORD"

The final promise is of freedom. Vindication means *exoneration, acquittal, or to clear of accusation, blame, suspicion, or doubt with supporting arguments or proof.* The Lord clears your name of accusation, blame, suspicion, and doubt. This is a promise that vindication is not from works of human hands but from the Lord Himself. He says, "from me, declares the LORD." I cannot think of anyone or anything else I want on my side as I face any battle. God might lead me into battle and ask me to fight, but my vindication comes from Him.

Rejoice in this day, the day that fear will no longer be a stronghold in your life. You may experience fear once in a while, but because of God's promises in Isaiah 54:13–17, God will not let it take root in you. If you have let fear take a hold of you, God won't let it stay. He will put you in situations that require you to face it and conquer it. He will ask you to put your faith into action. He won't do it for you, but as you do what He asks you to do and go where He asks you to go, He will fulfill His promise to remove fear from your life. It will be **"far removed"** as it says in Promise #5. This is how He works as father and son, or father and daughter. Now go and be healthy inside and out free from fear.

"Be strong and courageous, do not be afraid or discouraged, for the Lord God is with you wherever you go." (Joshua 1:9)

For Reflection:

Identify some strongholds of fearfulness in your life. What action will you take right now to overcome them?

_____

_____

Share a time in your life when you have *manifested what you feared*.

_____

_____

A LOVE LETTER

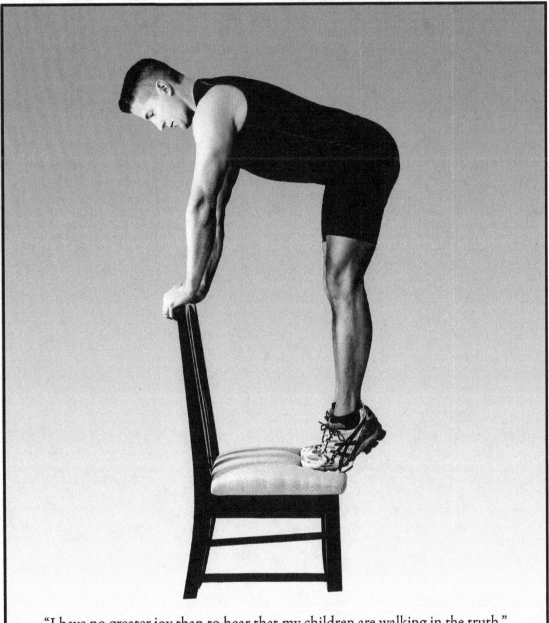

"I have no greater joy than to hear that my children are walking in the truth."
(3 John 1:4) "So there is hope for your future," declares the LORD.
"Your children (you) will return to their own land." (Jeremiah 31:17)

WEEK EIGHT

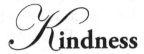

Kindness

*"An action displayed by both giving and receiving to ourselves
and others the gentleness of God"*

One day as I was lying in bed studying, I came across something amazing. I prayed about it constantly. It was about the true nature of God and how we are to live accordingly. As I discussed in the "Legalism" section in Week 4, a major problem in our world is that some people wrongfully project the judgment, anger, and wrath of God onto other people. Those of us who have experienced this atrocity have at times found it difficult to speak openly about God with people and have even found it difficult to believe in a God of anger and wrath. I have seen numerous people who have turned away from—and even run from—the church and their own faith in Christ because of religious abuse. It breaks my heart. What also breaks my heart is how few of us actually display one of the most distinguishing qualities of God, His loving kindness. Whether it came from the hand, or mouth of an abuser, or from our own negative view of ourselves, the pain and hurt can end now as we take to heart what Romans 2:1–4 tells us: **"You, therefore, have no excuse, you who pass judgment on someone else, for at whatever point you judge the other, you are condemning yourself, because you who pass judgment do the same things. Now we know that God's judgment against those who do such things is based on truth. So when you, a mere man, pass judgment on them and yet do the same things, do you think you will escape God's judgment? Or do you show contempt for the riches of his kindness, tolerance, and patience, not realizing that God's kindness leads you toward repentance?"**

I had read this before, but this time the last sentence jumped off the page at me: **"Or do you show contempt for the riches of his kindness, tolerance, and patience, not realizing that God's kindness leads you toward repentance?"** **This passage** reveals God's true nature and also shows how much He loves all of us. What is repentance? It is forgiveness with a change in action. But why would people want to change when they learn about how angry and disappointed God is in them? It says plainly here in Romans that it is the **"kindness of God that leads you to repentance,"** not anger, wrath, or judgment. There will be a day of judgment for everyone, but that is *not* what leads us toward repentance. It is kindness. Kindness is what makes a person hungry for the truth, hungry to know God intimately, and eager to change. How much resentment, contempt, and even hatred toward the church and faith in Christ have been created because of people's judgment, even your own judgment and condemning thoughts toward yourself? Our job is to love ourselves and others and show kindness, not judgment!

Oftentimes, a person's first experience of God is through a person showing **"kindness, tolerance and patience."** Showing kindness to people is how they first experience God's kindness. So often the kindness of God made manifest in our own lives is what leads others to repentance. Perhaps it has been difficult for you to ask forgiveness from God and other people for your unhealthy lifestyle because you have been afraid of judgment. If this has been your experience I can't say I blame you for not wanting to genuinely confess and change. But it is time to change by holding on to the kindness and gentleness of God's love. **Let His kindness lead you towards repentance!**

As ambassadors of Christ we are all called to manifest the loving-kindness of Jesus. Are we not called to love as He loved, to show kindness and gentleness to all we come in contact with? We spread the love and richness of Christ by loving others and ourselves! We may not love what a person does, but we are called to love and be kind to the person. Again, why would a person want to change if the God who is being crammed down their throats hates them? If you find yourself judging someone, it is probably out of pride, self-righteousness, or some kind of insecurity you have in yourself. Do not judge, but look into your own heart, remember the times you have fallen short, and be kind. Jesus was tortured and beaten beyond recognition, and while on the cross moments before His death, He looked at His captors and said, "Forgive them, Father, for they know not what they do." Jesus was kind, tolerant, and patient with the very people who were crucifying Him.

Your Closest Neighbor: You

Here is the clincher. How kind are you to *yourself*? How do you think of yourself—with confidence or insecurity, courage or fear, kindness or anger? Remember "the Great You Are"? What thoughts do you permit to tell you who *you are* or influence your decisions? How do you let people treat you—with respect and honor or with disrespect and dishonor? Being kind doesn't mean letting people walk all over you. Having a voice and standing up for yourself when violated in some way is very much a part of your heritage.

But let's get real for a moment. How do you really treat *yourself?*—with respect and honor, or disrespect and dishonor? How can you expect to ask forgiveness and change anything in your life if you view yourself as tainted and ugly? Are you walking free or are you stuck in the rut of guilt and shame and hence speaking and thinking awful things about yourself? Maybe you just feel whipped and beaten and think that is what you deserve. Tell Satan to kiss your entire $%@)*+$##!!! God wants all of us to live with His qualities flowing through us like rivers of running water. He wants us to own His truth for ourselves. He wants you to be kind to *yourself and others!* Being kind *to* yourself by receiving kindness *from* God is one of the most powerful forms of repentance. Forgiving yourself as God forgives you and being kind to yourself as God is kind "**leads you toward repentance.**" So many of us can't even look in a mirror without feeling shameful, insecure, weak, and timid, yet we shower others with a barrage of compliments, encouragements, and praises. If this is you, you must change this! I have encouraged so many women clients throughout my career to write on their mirrors with lipstick, "I AM beautiful" and "I AM worthy." I don't care if they don't initially feel it or even believe it. When they constantly say it, write it, and read it every day over and over they will eventually own it. And so will you if you are a woman reading this.

In essence, making healthy choices through exercise and nutrition begins by being kind to yourself. You must be kind to YOU! How much time do we spend every single week in the *Courage to Change Life Application Journal* learning how to change our thoughts, attitudes, and performances so they align with God's will for our life? True repentance is putting the TAP principle in alignment with God. Speak life and kindness in and over *yourself*, not just your family and loved ones. Remember that kindness is just as much an action as a thought or attitude. It is in our actions that kindness is evidenced in our lives, whether toward ourselves or others. Be kind to yourself and watch as God's kindness **"leads you toward repentance."**

Take a moment to digest the gentler side of kindness before moving on.

Much like cleaning an infected puncture wound in your child's leg by scrubbing it with soap and warm water and then disinfecting it with peroxide, or pulling a thorn from an animal's paw, kindness doesn't always feel good and it certainly doesn't always feel gentle. Once in college I took a pretty bad spill on my mountain bike, and one of the deep abrasions on my knee got badly infected. I went to the student health center on campus and watched in horror as the nurse used a stiff brush to scrub out the infection. Oh my goodness! The infection was right on the knee cap and she *reeeeeeally* scrubbed. Major pain! But after that, the infection was gone and it healed. Only a scar was left. This kind of tough love is also needed on a behavioral level to hold ourselves and others accountable for our actions. Why do we scold a child who runs into the street without looking and almost gets hit by a car? Because we want the child to be safe. But make no mistake, this form of kindness, though sometimes painful, is about love *not* judgment. If you approach a friend or family member about something that is harmful to him, or someone else, and in the process you shame, cause guilt, or condemn them for what they are doing, this is not kindness but judgment. As we teach or encourage people to change their behavior, we have a tremendous responsibility to come from a place of love. If they don't change right away, what does that have to do with you? Nothing! Just love them!

Though it doesn't always feel good as you exercise, you are being kind to yourself. It is no different from scrubbing the infection out of a wound. It is simply on the "preventive" side of kindness rather than the "treatment" side of kindness.

Talking to people about their health is no different. We must do it, but out of love. Before you can move on further with *Courage to Change*, you must again put the past behind you by asking for forgiveness and forgiving others. Being kind to yourself is the first step in making changes. Otherwise, the guilt and shame will paralyze you into taking no action at all.

> **Let God's loving kindness and gentleness lead you toward repentance so you can live in the freedom and power of positive life-change!**

Who do you know who needs help? Who do you know who could use more confidence and self-esteem? Many people are stuck in a vicious cycle in which their inability to stick to a program feeds their insecurities, which in turn feeds their inability to stick to a program. While they make changes, only God can conquer the fear and the shame. Let's all talk to others about being healthy. If you know someone who needs to make changes, send them to our website or give them a copy of this book, the *Life Application Journal, and the Captain's Log* as gifts and lovingly encourage them to get involved in *Courage to Change*, wherever they live! Help Silesia and I take back the health of this country, this world. Our families depend on it. Our lives depend on it and on *you* to spread the word.

As you will see in this week's lesson plan in the *Life Application Journal,* part of being kind to yourself is getting to know the little boy or girl in you and ministering to him or her. Your journal will walk you through the process. Have fun getting to know *you* and enjoy the wonderful process of being kind to yourself! Then watch how this filters into all of your other relationships.

For Reflection:

Name three things that you do to love and take care of yourself (being kind to your closest neighbor—you)?

_____

_____

What are three ways you can minister to the little boy or girl inside of you?

_____

_____

Conquering Shame

"Living in freedom by putting the past behind you"

Early in my career in Denver in 1998, I had the rare privilege of working with Julie, a young woman who really wanted change. One day as I was in the facility getting ready to train a client, she came up to me, and with some reluctance and fear, told me that she needed my help to lose weight. She was 24 years old and weighed approximately 227 pounds. She was very active in "Young Life" and loved the Lord. She was waiting until marriage to have sex and seemed in many ways to be on track in her Christian walk. But there was something missing. She had no comprehension of the "as yourself" part of **"love your neighbor as yourself."** In fact she loathed herself, hated who she had become, and viewed herself as a fat, unattractive, and an unapproachable woman. For over two years I trained her. We went through tears, intense emotions, and even that love-hate relationship I often get from clients as I challenge them. We became very close, and together we tackled fear, feelings of inadequacy, unworthiness, and insecurity.

I remember one exercise I did with her that surprised both of us. She was dealing with so much negativity and hopelessness that it drained her and sometimes even *me*. So as we trained one afternoon at our normal time of 1:00, I asked her to trust me before we started the next exercise. She agreed to trust me, not knowing what I was going to do. I asked her to hold five-pound weights out to her side for as long as she could. But while she did this, she had to repeat over and over, "I am fat and ugly! I am fat and ugly!" She looked at me with those same eyes I usually got as I challenged her, but she did what I asked. She struggled and struggled with her strength and pushed herself until her shoulders gave out. After a few minutes of rest, we repeated the exercise, only this time I asked her to say with power and authority, "I am strong and beautiful! I am strong and beautiful!" Her entire countenance changed. As she fought fatigue, I continued to encourage her to actually mean what she was saying and to say it more and more loudly as she went on. By the time she reached total muscle fatigue the second time, she had more than doubled her time of holding up the weights. And this was after her muscles had already been fatigued from her previous set. She learned that day that her physical energy, strength, and endurance were in direct proportion to her mental state and to how her thoughts and attitudes were in alignment with God. She amazed herself, and as we trained, each day was more empowering than the day before. I watched her go from a scared, insecure little girl to a mature, confident, beautiful young woman. In the first year she lost 75 pounds. She went from 227 to 152 pounds and was no longer exercising because of her need to lose weight or out of insecurity and hopelessness. She was exercising because she loved it. She frequently ran 5K races and competed in mini-triathlons. She did this when she was still 60 pounds overweight. As she went skiing with her friends, she would ski circles around everyone all day long because of the physical endurance she had gained through our training. And these were friends who used to ski circles around her.

I was so proud of her. She began to inspire me, and at times when I would feel like stopping during a workout, I would think of her and her determination and *Courage to Change,* and I would press on. But all this time as we trained and went through all this life-change, she was still holding onto something....

Every time I asked her if I could use a "before and after" picture to inspire others in my marketing, she would clam up and make excuses and sometimes her attitude was short, abrupt, and even arrogant. When she first came to me she had no self-esteem, no confidence, and no self-worth other than her job and relationship with God. She had become the exact opposite. What I mean by that is this: In my life I have often found something to be true, even with myself. A person will often go to extremes before striking a balance in all areas of his or her life. Once a person figures out how to change, he often goes too far in the other direction in an attempt to get as far away from the "old person" as possible. I could see this happening to her. I was proud every day for her progress, but I also was discerning enough to know that she hadn't yet found balance or peace in her heart regarding her past.

For a while she became very controlling, and many of my colleagues and I noticed it. That control was serving to keep her from truly moving forward in her life. I am talking about her entire life, the life of a beautiful young woman who still viewed herself as a fat little girl. That control issue contributed to her inability to let go of the past. She was living in shame.

I understood why and knew that it was perfectly natural to go from one extreme to the other, but it was time for her to hear it from me. It was time for her to conquer her shame. I actually offered to train her for free for a while if she let me use her "before" picture. My decision to make her that offer was based on helping her relinquish her control of her past and the control she felt she must have in the present. If that helped me get more clients, great, but it wasn't why I wanted to do it. I had plenty of clients. Her unwillingness to give up her controlling past was fueling her desire to control everything around her.

She kept bringing up the word *privacy* in describing her reasons for not letting me use her picture in my promotional material. I was sensitive to that and even prayed about it, but I felt that there was an underlying reason she refused to let me use the picture. I felt deep inside that her reasons were fear-based excuses keeping her from relinquishing the control her past had over her.

I remember sharing with her that because of her past, she felt as though everyone was out to get her and would take advantage of her. Why? A person who is insecure is an easy target for manipulation and being taken advantage of. Deep down, she wanted so badly to avoid being manipulated again that she looked for it all around her. That was where her controlling tendencies came from. Most of her life she hadn't been able to control her weight and habits, so she had to control everything else around her. That was the extreme I was talking about earlier. That intense determination to never be manipulated again was evidence that her past fear and shame were still controlling her present life. It was a natural progression and process to her putting the past behind her, but it still needed to change.

I understood exactly where she was. When I lived in Dallas the first time before moving to Denver, I constantly looked for people who were trying to take advantage of me. Coming from a small town in western Kansas, I was somewhat naive and an easy target. I later learned that actually looking out for people who might take advantage of me was a way of living my life with resentment and a victim mentality, both toward the people who might try to control me and toward myself for the naiveté I used to live in. Peace does not result from this kind of thinking!

My client was seeking balance, a godly balance and freedom from her past. But I could sense the tremendous amount of pressure she put on herself. Without the pressure and control, she felt weak and powerless, and it reminded her of where she used to be. She needed to embrace her past and let God use it to strengthen her. But it was very important for her to be careful not to confuse resentment with strength because that was where she was residing. I frequently told her to spend some time alone with God and ask Him to help her embrace her past. For her to ask Him to take that which she hungered and thirsted for out of her life so that her desires resulted in a peaceful heart. I also recommended that she ask God for the wisdom to recognize and overcome the behaviors that held her back.

As I shared my concerns with her, she responded at times with cold, crass, and very defensive remarks, all of which was perfectly natural. I shared with her a theory I had. As I did, I reminded her that my goal was to help her conquer the shame she was living in. I also reminded her that she was stuck with me for the rest of her life! And she is!

In my theory, I posed five main questions, which eventually uncovered the truth about her embarrassment in exposing her past weight problem. These are the questions I asked and my commentary that went with them.

Question 1

Did she still have a difficult time with her past?

Of course she did, which was fine, for a while. But what was it about her life that kept her from her future?

Question 2

Did she feel shame because of her past weight problem?

I believed so and knew she was working on that. I had been there every step of the way trying to support her in overcoming that shame. But what was it about having her picture on some promotional material that could possibly be fueling that feeling of shame? I encouraged her to please read on.

Question 3

Is it up to you to overcome this shame and embarrassment of being heavy in your past?

Of course it was, she and God working together. No one could deal with this except her. But what is one possible reason she held on so tightly to her past, afraid of being seen as a fat little girl, which she wasn't! Who had she been hiding from?

Question 4

Why might she have such a problem with a picture of her being shown with other clients outside the club?

I believed she wasn't as concerned about what strangers would say when they saw where she used to be as she was about what someone close to her would say if and when that person found out the "BIG SECRET." This led to my final question.

Question 5

Had she told her boyfriend about how far she had come?

This was a very serious question, and I knew that the answer was *no, she hadn't!* She was so afraid that if he went out somewhere and saw her picture, he wouldn't love her anymore. If that was the man she was to marry, the relationship should begin with trust and honesty, not shame, fear, and distrust. If he was a loving man, knowing how far she had come would only make him love her that much more. Secrets are not the foundation of any relationship. I believed in my heart that this was a paramount factor in her growth, the final hurdle. Her heart was so afraid of rejection that it consumed her. By being afraid her boyfriend would reject her, she had already been rejected. That kind of fear will eventually surface in all of our relationships. If that man was worth her time, she might very well offend him by keeping it from him. If he was a great guy worthy of her time, she needed to trust in him and believe in his ability to be her biggest supporter in life. If she could not trust him, then it wasn't fair to either one of them, and maybe she wasn't with the right man.

I was so proud of her, not simply because she had lost the weight but because of her drive, determination, and that work *she* had done to accomplish it. That was the most attractive aspect about her whole story. The person she had become was so awesome and inspiring. The man in her life should love her drive, determination, accomplishments, and desire to be the best she could be. And he should also love her body because it was beautiful. Sharing with him her accomplishments would only give him reason to love her that much more. I remember telling her, "If it doesn't inspire him, he's not worth your time. Bye-bye!" I also talked to her about how important physical chemistry was in a relationship. And in saying that, I asked her if she had looked in the mirror lately. She was drop-dead gorgeous. She was truly a beautiful young woman. But she had to believe that for herself!

Secrets based on shame paralyze you in relation to a godly spirit and make it impossible for you to see yourself through God's eyes. God is not ashamed of you, so why should you be? True forgiveness or repentance of any behavior comes with absolutely no memory of the past other than that which reminds you of where God has delivered you from. God is oh so proud of you!

> "Yet if you devote your heart to him and stretch out your hands to him, if you put away the sin that is in your hand and allow no evil to dwell in your tent, then you will lift up your face without shame; you will stand firm and without fear. You will surely forget your trouble, recalling it only as waters gone by. Life will be brighter than noonday, and darkness will become like morning. You will be secure, because there is hope; you will look about you and take your rest in safety. You will lie down, with no one to make you

afraid, and many will court your favor." (Job 11:13–19)

During one of our sessions, a friend of mine saw us together. He thought she was beautiful and asked me about her. So I told him a brief history of our road together and the goals she had surpassed. Once I told him, he was even more amazed by her. He too became instantly inspired and commented on how awesome she was. He then proceeded to ask me if she was single and told me that I should be going after her. He said this not because of her accomplishments but because he really did think she was beautiful. The point was that he didn't care where she used to be—he found her entire story beautiful and inspiring. What she had accomplished *was* indeed beautiful. The woman she had become and was becoming was beautiful. Physically, she was beautiful and attracted the attention of a number of men (not that that was her goal). They liked what they saw, **"and many will court your favor."** But even after losing more than 100 pounds, she internally and subconsciously still saw herself as a fat little girl. It was time she stopped living a lie and started seeing herself as *beautiful.* I told her to stand up, raise her arms over her head, and say out loud five times every day, "I AM BEAUTIFUL!" I told her to smile from ear to ear and love herself enough to be honest and open to those around her. No more secrets. I told her to accept who she was—a beautiful, young, attractive woman—and to peacefully breathe the air God gave her; to be thankful and gracious for her life.

Taking off the weight took time and a lot of healing, but relinquishing the control the past had over her was the final step that would change her life. Only then could she finally see herself for who she really was—a beautiful, lean, intelligent, godly woman.

It was during her struggle with overcoming shame that I moved from Denver back to Dallas as part of my own growth and *Courage to Change.* It was difficult to leave her and all of my clients because of how intimate our relationships were. A couple of years passed before one day I felt compelled to write her an e-mail to see how she was doing. She replied with one of her usual jokes—saying she had put all of her weight back on and then some. She hadn't, of course, and was still living according to the *Courage to Change* principles I taught her and still loved competing in local triathlons in Denver. I really enjoyed getting caught up. It was like a single day hadn't gone by.

It turned out that after a year-and-a-half courtship she finally mustered the courage to break up with the boyfriend she had had during the time I was there. I don't know whether or not she ever told him the details of her "heavy" past. But sharing her past with him terrified her. After she broke up with him Julie had time to literally get comfortable in her new skin! I could tell as I talked to her that she just needed time. She had to go through some hard times to break free from her old mentality, but she did it with God as her rock. God parted the sea and she had to walk through it. She is doing amazing things. Being willing to do the work and persevere through the hard stuff, she now owns her own business with offices spread throughout the country, still lives in the freedom of a lean healthy lifestyle, and is loved by friends and family. God restored her abundantly more than she could have ever imagined!

Julie will tell you that even though she is proud of herself for all of her accomplishments, she still deals with her body image every day. She is continuing to practice taking her thoughts and attitudes and making them obedient to Christ, and seeing herself through His eyes, not her own. Practicing the TAP Principle and I AM Declaration is something she will do for the rest of her life. So, how do we know that she, with God's help, conquered the shame in her life? Because she is able and willing to tell her story in the hopes that it will help free some of you from your own shame. Her past is no longer about "her", it is about YOU!

Julie's Testimony:

November 2, 2009

A little history. I was a chubby child, turned fat teenager, turned obese adult. Interestingly enough, so was my mother. I lost all of my weight in my early 20s, and another interesting fact, so did my mom. We both had the difficult and wonderful experience of losing the weight and blooming late to discover our true beauty.

Please understand that in my formative years I was loved more than any child could be loved. I had experiences and opportunities that only a privileged few get. My home was a very safe and happy haven. My parents set an amazing example of love, work ethic and faith and gave me a sister that is the most remarkable woman you could hope to meet and one whom I would be incomplete without. Yet, despite all this, lonely and quietly I struggled. Regardless how rosy our childhood was we all have struggles. This happens to be my struggle.

I think my mom was so scared that I would carry the same burdens and sadness that result from being a fat child and teenager that she did everything she knew how to do to prevent that from happening to a daughter she loved so dearly. She loved and loves me more than she loves herself and wanted to protect me from the wounds and scars from a fat childhood. Thus food was "bad" in my household. Snacking was the enemy, and breakfast was never encouraged. Of course we now know that these dieting tips will sabotage your metabolism, but back then this was the message, and my mother and I heard it loud and clear. The doctors said "No snacking!" So no snacking it was. I would skip breakfast and lunch, not snack all day, and then come home from school and sports STARVING. Then I would binge eat from 5:00 p.m. until bedtime. This went on from junior high until I was 24.

Inside I was miserable, ashamed and quietly dying. But no one knew that because outside I was happy, gregarious and always laughing. *What a lie!* Why, you ask? Because I believed that if I admitted to others how unhappy the weight made me they would judge me for choosing to do nothing about it or, worse, shame me for my unwillingness to make hard changes and real sacrifices. Instead of admitting that hard truth, I took the other road: I *acted* as though I was happy and settled into the unhappy realization that being "heavy" was simply who I was. Then I had my "Ah Ha" moment.

My younger sister, gorgeous inside and out, got engaged. She asked me to be her Maid of Honor and requested that I pick the Bridesmaid dresses. She knew that dress shopping was going to be an uncomfortable ordeal (to say the least—at that time I was wearing a size 20). We searched high and low and ended up having the dresses custom made. At this stage in my life and my cycle of weight gain, it was a very rare moment when I felt good about myself. But on the day of my sister's wedding I actually felt great! I loved my dress and I was so proud to stand by my sister's side. Then came the lightning bolt. Six weeks after the wedding, the photographer's proofs arrived. There I was in hundreds of photos. FAT! I looked like I weighed 227 pounds. Because I *did*. The shame was so great I could barley breathe, and the tears wouldn't stop. I looked like what the scale said and the scale did not lie. And that was it. Something snapped. Changed. Catapulted. FOREVER.

The next day, after sobbing uncontrollably over those proofs, I walked into the Cherry Creek Sporting Club and met Brian Wellbrock. Brian and I had an instant connection spiritually and at the core. He saw my pain and knew my story before any words were exchanged. We trained together for the next two-and-a-half years, and it went like this: Monday, Wednesday and Friday—resistance training with Brian (and the hardest work I have ever done) from 1:00-2:00; Cardio on my own from 2:00-2:30. Tuesday, Thursday and Saturday—one hour of Cardio on my own. Every week for two-and-a-half years! Faithfully!

When I finished my time with Brian I was 152 pounds. I had lost 75 pounds! As I am writing this 12years later I am 152 pounds. Ironic? I don't think so…. I have been back up as high as 167 and have been as low as 137 (running 5 days a week and perfect on my nutrition), but my body has a new normal and thankfully it is not 227. My new, or not so new, normal (it's been 12 years) is a size 10 and always right around 150 pounds, give or take five pounds. The great thing about this new normal is that I do not have to train at the excruciating levels I originally did to lose such a significant amount of weight. I eat a healthy, balanced diet (mostly) and when I overindulge or slip, I just think, tomorrow is a new day and I will do better.

I go through phases where I really get after it and will train for a half marathon (to date I have run five) and then I will slow it down for a few months and walk on the treadmill three times a week or hike with the dog. Either way, I never adjust up or down more than five or so pounds because it is no longer about the weight. It's about being healthy, balanced and authentic! Now the giggles are real and the smile is true!

It would be unfair and impossible to summarize in a page what Brian and I accomplished together in those painful moments in and out of the gym, so I will end on this. I thank God for placing Brian in my life at a time when I needed him most and I thank you, Brian Wellbrock. Thank you for every bead of sweat, every tear, every heated word, every mile, every lunge, every curl, every pound, and every inch. I thank you. Everyone needs someone at some time in their lifetime and I desperately needed Brian at this chapter in my life. We did it the right way. We did it the hard way, and the hard way is what made it great.

Today I live in Montana and know love, laughter and life to the fullest. I wish you my kind of success.

---Julie

Meet Julie!

Beautiful at 227 pounds

Beautiful at 136 pounds

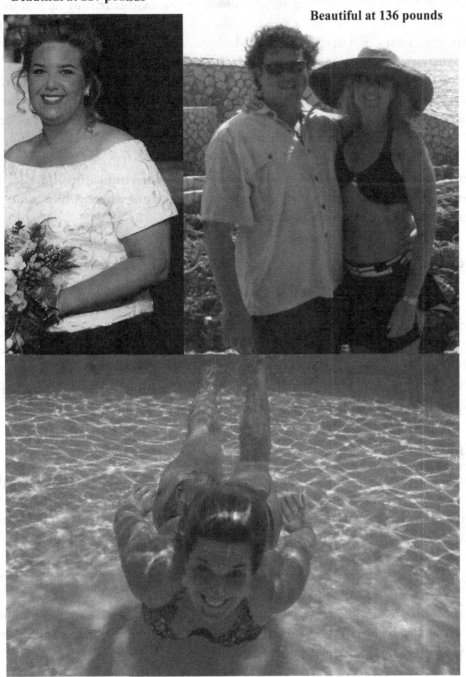

Beautiful at 150 pounds and free! Her smile says it all!
Julie finally realized she didn't lose her weight to make herself MORE beautiful!
She lost her weight BECAUSE SHE WAS AND IS beautiful!
Like Julie does in this picture, tell shame to take a flying leap off a tall cliff!

Friends, freedom from your past is not something that just I want for you, it is something God longs for you to walk in. I know you want it as well. Freedom from your past does not take anything away from who you were. It simply means not letting it control your emotions and actions. If I asked you to submit a before-and-after picture, would you be able to send it without shame? You know how shame shows up in your life. It may look different to each of us, but it must be dealt with in order for you to be free in your walk with God. Shame may show up from a failed marriage or even a past drug addiction. Maybe you stayed in an abusive relationship too long and feel shame for not getting out sooner. Maybe you feel shame because you haven't spent enough time with your children and work too much. Whatever it is, focus on your love affair with Christ and remember, **"Therefore, there is now no condemnation for those who are in Christ Jesus"** (Romans 8:1). Change what you need to change about your life and heal from the hurts, but let God put your past behind you where it belongs.

> **Even if you have confessed and changed your actions of an unhealthy lifestyle, if you can not openly and freely profess your testimony of where you've come from, then you are not truly free from it!**

The Gift of Your Testimony

Just remember that so many people's inspiration comes from people like you who have overcome, or are in the process of conquering, their weight issue, no matter how big or small the starting point was. Whatever a person is going through, it is important that he or she can go to someone like you, who has gone through it, for help and support. That is why ultimately this book and journal series works best in group settings within churches, businesses, health facilities, universities, family get-togethers, and Bible studies. **I truly believe that every person who shares his or her story will, without a doubt, save at least one person's life through testimony.**

Three things...

Your testimony is a gift to others! Freedom comes when you are able to freely and willingly give that testimony away. Anytime a gift is given, three things must happen. And when they do, shame will be a thing of the past. First, the gift must be crucified or freely given away (the meaning of the crucifixion). Second, the gift must be buried. This means to wash your hands of it and have no expectations of earning a return on your gift. Third, one must bear witness to the resurrection of what your gift produced (the harvest if you will). Bearing witness to the harvest means witnessing the changes in yourself and others based on what you have freely given—what your gift gave birth to. This pertains to any gift, whether it is to yourself, to someone else, or to a combination of both, which most gifts are. Your testimony is a gift, and those three things must happen for you to find your freedom. Be free and walk confidently into your future!

"Anyone who trusts in him will never be put to shame." (Romans 10:11)

For Reflection:

Shame is a "secret killer." In the space below, write down something that you have done that you are ashamed of and, once it is outside of you, give it to God, accept His forgiveness, and let it go.

_____

_____

Share your testimony—emphasizing not "how bad you were" but "how great God is."

_____

_____

CONQUERING CONTROL and ADDICTION

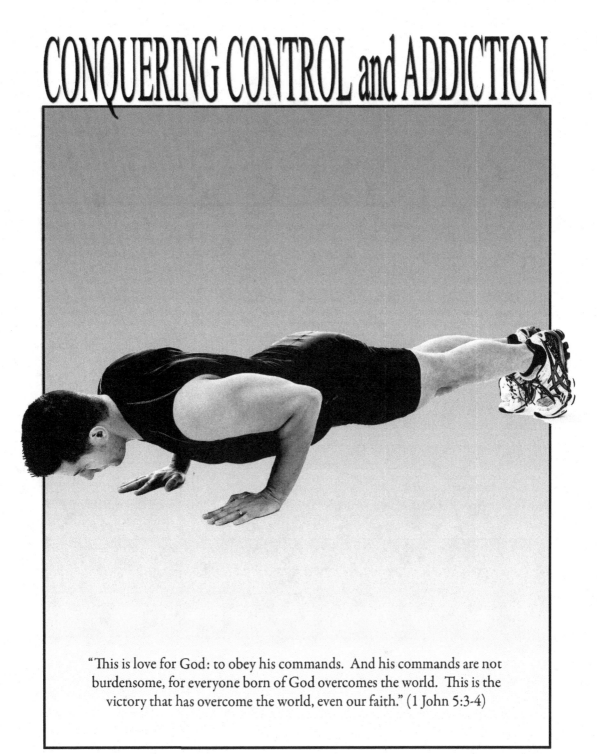

"This is love for God: to obey his commands. And his commands are not burdensome, for everyone born of God overcomes the world. This is the victory that has overcome the world, even our faith." (1 John 5:3-4)

WEEK NINE

Hunger and Thirst

The things we desire often turn into vices, crutches, addictions, obsessions, or thirst and hunger. Anything that controls, or has the potential to control you, is a thirst or hunger. We must learn to identify the things we hunger and thirst for. First, I want you to know that giving things up is not part of this program, nor should it be. Anything you give up or try to give up will control you. Now, bear with me. I am not saying swear off pizza and forsake bacon ever after or to stay away from bread for the rest of your life. I am not saying give up chocolate cake either. What I *am* saying is that you need to relinquish the control these items have *over you*.

If you give up smoking and yet do nothing to take the hunger or thirst for smoking out of your life, it will still control you. Do you think of yourself as an ex-smoker or a nonsmoker? If you refer to yourself as an ex-smoker, chances are that you "quit smoking" instead of changed your thought patterns and behavior to that of a nonsmoker. Though you quit smoking, you may still hunger for it and are still enslaved by its control over you. Remember the I AM! "I am a nonsmoker!" Period! And say it with authority!

Your hunger and thirst for something is equally important as the act of giving it up. Think of money. You certainly aren't going to give up making money if it controls you. But when you relinquish the control money has over you, you are free from its bondage. You may go on to make even more money because you give it to God and let Him control *it* rather than allow *it* to control you. It all comes back to the hunger and thirst for something and the reasons for that hunger and thirst. As you learned earlier, you will begin to change your desires (of the flesh and the world) to those "of the Father." And when this happens as you surrender to Christ in everything:

"Never again will you hunger, never again will you thirst." (Revelation 7:16)

Rather than thinking of yourself as giving up certain foods while losing weight, simply look at it as a conscious decision to refrain from those foods for a while until you get yourself under control and reach your goals. When it is time to maintain your current fitness goals as far as body fat goes, you can moderately integrate all kinds of foods back into your life. But the control will be *yours*—not the food's! Now, if your hunger or thirst is for drugs or alcohol, then you need to make that decision final and continue to work on eliminating the desires and acts altogether.

Don't simply quit smoking! Ask for the strength and conviction to no longer do something that is harmful to yourself and others. Don't just quit eating unhealthy food. Ask God to help give you a hunger for healthy food. Don't just start exercising because you have to. Ask God for the *hunger* to make yourself strong and vibrant. Don't just stop doing drugs. Ask God to deliver you from the control they have over you and to take your thirst and hunger for them away. **Most other programs don't work over the long haul because only Jesus Christ can deliver you, or**

free you, from the oppression of negative or destructive behaviors. As you turn to Him, the only thing you should hunger and thirst for is Him.

"Blessed are those who hunger and thirst for righteousness." (Matthew 5:6)

As you learned earlier, destructive thoughts, attitudes, and behaviors lead you into a downward spiral of low self-esteem, unworthiness, shame, and condemnation. It is impossible to be at your best if your perception of yourself, your physical image of yourself, is tainted. Regaining this authority and overcoming these behaviors means that there are things you have no control over and other things that you do have control over. The things you *do* have control over (by your actions) dictate in large part how you view yourself.

Example: If the topic is weight, there are things you do and do not have control over. If a woman is pregnant, of course she is going to gain some weight, which is a natural progression that helps protect the unborn child. Since this, within reason, is out of her control, there is absolutely no reason to let it affect her confidence. But if a person lets herself go and gains a lot of weight for various reasons that are in fact controllable, the result is a feeling of unattractiveness that slowly strips her of her confidence.

Another example is this: Let's say that every time a person has a bad day, he decides to eat a pizza and two bowls of ice cream. He has thus created an emotional attachment to food rather than going to God and dealing directly with the problems causing that attachment.

Many of you have low self-esteem. You may have had some bad experiences that render you, at least in your own eyes, less desirable. This in turn has caused you to feel unattractive, and this feeling has a direct impact on your self-confidence. What often happens is that you go into denial of the fact that your perception of your own physical attractiveness affects your confidence, so you don't break the negative pattern. Whether the problem is alcoholism, an eating disorder, drugs, pornography, cursing, envy, or a weight problem, denial plays a huge part in keeping the problem alive.

My Own Addiction

I battle with those same things all the time. I have taken my body to an extreme, having had only 2% body fat in one of my body building competitions. When I returned to a healthier body fat percentage, I felt fat. I actually dealt with the opposite of anorexia, a problem called *muscle dysmorphia*. This is actually a psychological term used to describe a person's obsession with and addiction to muscle growth and being muscular to feel important or noticed. There were times in college I would do push-ups before entering a room of people because I felt more confident in myself if I had "a pump." I actually felt more worthy of being there if I was bigger. Though I competed in body building drug free (steroid free), there were a few times I actually took steroids in an attempt to better myself. What a lie! I actually believed that there were two kinds of people who took steroids. One person would do it for a power kick and anger fix, and the other (like me) would do it as an athlete simply trying to better himself. What a joke! I finally heard God telling me that I was better than that and that it was wrong. At the time, my hunger for size and strength did not come from God but from the world. *I once was blind, but now I see!* Christ delivered me from the vanity of exercise and showed me how to be healthy and fit *His* way. I have never been the same since. It has been beautiful. Now I know what is healthy and what isn't but still must be careful not to regress. So we have to be careful not to get vain—but the feeling of attractiveness isn't vanity. It is a beautiful, God-given right!

So where did the root of my addiction originate? As I learned about my behavior from pastors and counselors and looked to God for both giving and receiving forgiveness, I began getting to the root of the addictive behavior that had controlled me.

I grew up in an alcoholic family. My dad would come home after work and down a case of Coors every night. I vowed never to be like that. And I didn't. Instead of becoming an alcoholic, I became a workaholic, workout-aholic, and perfectionist. Though I didn't drink alcohol, I still took on a spirit of addiction. Many of you who have tried to quit smoking have gained *a lot* of weight. Why? Because your problem isn't smoking, it is addiction. As you quit smoking, your addiction simply got transferred to something else—from tobacco to food.

My behavior was a spiritual root of addiction, so just because I didn't drink, I expressed the behavior in other ways. I had to be the best in everything or I didn't feel worthy. I didn't miss a single workout in over nine years! Some of you think that is impressive. Let me ask you a question. How hard is it to do something you are addicted to? It isn't! It is easy! Take away the addiction and I will show you a completely different person. I now must base my exercise on a covenant with God because my addiction has been lifted. God keeps me in check on a daily basis, but some days are strictly based on commitment. Now that the spirit of addiction has been lifted, I have those days where I really don't want to exercise. But I do it anyway out of my love for God and the covenant I made with Him to be healthy. Not to mention the commitment I made to my wife, Silesia, as I said my marriage vows "In sickness or in health!" I choose health, not just for me, but for her because I love her and want to honor her with good health! You do have a choice you know!

So how did I beat it? Recall that in the section on fear we said that *what we fear, we manifest.* I made a vow never to be like my dad, but what happened was that because my vow was made out of fear, I became just like him. It just looked different. He was addicted to beer, I was addicted to work, working out and being "perfect," typical for an ACOA (Adult Child Of an Alcoholic). As I grew in my love affair with Christ, He showed me forgiveness toward my dad and showed me the areas I needed to change and let go. I found that as I longed for God, there was no room in my life for worldly stuff. My addictions were simply "fixes" or false securities, and as I let God in and felt His amazing love, He took their place. **Nothing I was ever addicted to felt as good as the love of God!** God took me through the four levels of obedience in each area of my life, helped me change my thoughts, attitudes, and performance (TAP), and taught me how to own His truth found in the Bible ("I Am"). He taught me perseverance, true commitment free from addiction, and the power of forgiveness. He got my priorities to line up in the proper order (Week 11) and showed me how to love myself. I see a Christian counselor, get mentored and held accountable by my pastor and go to church services and seminars.

Control and addiction is simply man's attempt to feel the presence of God by worldly means. Whether you have a chemical dependency, food addiction, people-pleaser addiction, anger addiction, fear addiction, envy addiction, jealousy addiction, lust or pornography addiction, sex addiction, wealth addiction, health addiction, power addiction, gambling addiction, or shoe

Courage to Change

addiction, it is the enemy's trickery deceiving you into believing that you will get the same "high" you would get from surrendering your life to Christ. But it is all a lie! There is no greater feeling in the world than the love of God running through you like rivers of running water. Freedom is the goal of Christ. Bondage is the goal of addiction.

What are you addicted to?

Fear	Drama
Food	Television
Alcohol	Fitness
Drugs	Success
People pleasing	Being right
Anger	Acceptance
Envy	Gambling
Jealousy	Failure
Lust or pornography	Power
Sex	Wealth

All of the lies in the "I Am" declaration are potential addictions. Addiction of any kind will always be made manifest in your physical actions (your behavior). I have talked about the addiction present in my work earlier in *Courage to Change*. Again, it was my attempt to feel the presence of God by worldly means. It didn't work. Local and national recognition, television and radio appearances, a huge client base, and being more muscular than most professional athletes felt pretty good.

So why did I keep trying to do more and more? Why did I work 55-hour weeks and never let myself have any fun outside of work? Because my value came from addiction and not from God.

224

And it was never enough. It couldn't fulfill me no matter how far I went. That lifestyle fried me. So I let it all go. Again, I unknowingly believed the lie that those things would ultimately make me feel as good as God's love. God may take me to a place where I receive that kind of recognition again, but it will not have anything to do with me or what gives me value. It will be about Him and bringing glory to *His* name not mine!

I would challenge all of you to embrace the concept or theory that addiction is nothing more than **man's attempt to feel the presence of God by worldly means, a Holy Spirit quick fix.** It is a lie from the enemy trying to keep you from truly knowing the powerful deliverance that comes from a love affair with Jesus Christ. Let God into your heart right now and let him rid you of the world because nothing the world has to offer will make you feel as good and as worthy as God's love does. **"And blessed be God Most High, who delivered your enemies into your hand"** (Genesis 14:20). When you truly know this, even the feeling won't matter. You will simply know it!

All of you battling some kind of addiction know that it takes time and hard work. Addiction usually stems from a deeper root, a way for you to fill a void from something missing in your life. What is usually missing is…*God*. Sure, we sometimes long for our mother or father to tell us they love us when their actions may not support this. Sure, we miss the support of people who should be supporting us. But even that love and support we may or may not receive can't touch the amazing love and intimacy that comes with Christ. Nothing—and I mean *nothing*—else comes close. Go to the source to be in God's presence, God himself, and live free from the lies that come with addiction.

Jesus is everything you will ever need and is the only drug you will ever get high on again!

For Reflection:

Identify the most destructive addiction (or two) in your life. What void are you trying to fill with the addiction?

_____

_____

Can God fill that void? Ask Him to do so now and watch (observe) for love notes in the days to come as He does so. Make a note of them when they come in your *Life Application Journal.*

_____

_____

Character

"An account of the Christ-like qualities or peculiarities of a person"

One of the goals of *Courage to Change* is to develop and nurture your Christ-like character. Control by and addiction to anything in this world keeps you from developing this kind of character. The following story is a beautiful example of how we develop a strong Christ-like character. The setting is a stormy summer evening on the Gulf Coast of eastern Texas.

The clouds rolled in, the sun began to fade, and the stadium lights came on as Matthew, our 11-year-old (at the time), prepared for the 200 meter dash at the Texas Amateur Athlete Federation regional track meet in Texas City in the summer of 2006. The heat of the day was past and in its place was an ominous black sky, fitting for the events that would follow. It was 9:30 p.m., and he was yet to run his race. He had already struggled a little in the 100 meter dash and long jump, taking fourth place in the 100 and fifth in the long jump. He had been a little off, and the competition was much fiercer than at his last state qualifier meet a month prior. But he kept his cool, brushed himself off, and mentally prepared himself for the 200. Finally, it was time. His heat came up, he was placed in his lane, and he knelt down to get in position for the gun to go off. We marveled at how many amazing athletes were in the competition. His opponents looked serious and *huge*. He was running against 11 and 12 year olds, some of them sporting mustaches.

The whistle sounded, the gun went up, and *BAM!* they were off. We had been working on how to hug the curve and run smoothly and gracefully. As he rounded the curve, he looked amazing. He was smooth and graceful, he hugged the curve like a champion, and his stride was long and fast. He quickly took the lead and kept it. Not only did he keep it, he pulled farther away from everyone in his heat throughout the entire race, beating the second-place finisher by almost two seconds. The other heats were super fast. We prayed that his first-place time would still make it in the top three overall, sending him to the state track meet in Round Rock, Texas, two weeks later.

As we awaited announcement of the overall results, we noticed some commotion down by the tent in the infield, the nerve center of the place where everything is run and announced. Matthew and his coach were there talking to the officials and another runner. Matthew looked frustrated and concerned. He had tied a runner in a different heat for the third-place spot. Yes, the exact same time. The officials weren't sure what to do. They suggested flipping a coin, but Matthew (shy, soft-spoken Matthew) spoke up and protested. He wanted to run again. The other kid didn't want to and was intimidated by the whole thing. But Matthew didn't relent. He absolutely insisted that they run again. One of the officials agreed with him saying, "Going to state is not based on the luck of a coin-toss but on the performance of each runner." So there you have it. Matthew would have to wait for the entire track meet to be over to have his run-off. Remember, it had already been a long day and was approaching 10:00 p.m., his usual bedtime in the summer. But he didn't look frazzled at all. **He would rather run the race again and lose than win with a coin-toss and go to state!** (read that again) **He would rather run the race again and lose than win with a coin-toss and go to state!** He wanted to *earn* it! I was so proud of him, I couldn't stand it. So we went back in the stands and rested and strategized. The other runner had an amazing start, better than Matthew in the first race. So I told him he would need to come off the start fast and aggressively and turn on his "nitro" throughout the entire race. He drank some Gatorade, took off his shoes, and kept his confident eyes on the other runner, still on the infield by the tent. He still didn't want to run again. Matthew just studied him like an eagle scouting its prey. His eyes were sharp, confident, and *in the zone.*

About an hour later, between 10:30 and 10:45, the meet was over and it was time for the run-off. The official told the runners that they would be running in lanes 2 and 3. Matthew looked at the other runner and told him to choose. The runner's father who was there was a bit surprised at Matthew's confidence and even commented on it. The other runner chose the inside lane. I said a few exciting words of encouragement, and after making sure that the track was cleared, Matthew and his opponent got in their starting positions. All of our hearts were pounding and about to jump out of our chests with excitement and anticipation. I ran over to the finish line so I could see them finish. The whistle blew, the gun went up, and *BAM!* they were off.

Matthew took the lead early with the most amazing start. He turned his "nitro" on from the very beginning and pulled ahead as they rounded the curve. His stride was long and fast and his arms pumped like mad. He ran so smoothly that you could barely see his head move. But as they came around the corner, the other runner had a kick and passed Matthew. The next 50 meters, the other runner kept pulling ahead and looked as if he would clinch the race. But Matthew had other plans. He had already won the race in his mind before he actually ran it. All of a sudden came a second burst of "nitro," and with only 50 meters left, Matthew came back neck-to-neck with his opponent. I was screaming. Silesia was screaming. Our daughter Shelby and everyone in the stands were screaming as they approached the finish line. In those last 50 meters, they must have changed from first to second four times. At the finish line, the other runner seemed to pull ahead just a bit, but out of nowhere Matthew leaned his whole body forward, like a professional athlete would in the Olympics. How did he know how to do that? We had never worked on "the lean" before.

Guess what? Another photo finish. The clock did not operate in milliseconds and gauged them as having the *exact same time* again. Both boys completed the race a whole second faster than in their earlier first race. Had they run that time in the first race, both would be going to state. So we all went to the tent and watched as the officials rewound the tape and replayed it at least ten times. Once again a small group formed as we viewed the tape again and again. The foot of the other runner actually passed the finish line first, but they don't go by feet but by the body. As the officials leaned in and studied the somewhat blurry photo finish, they could make out a shoulder crossing the finish line first. It was Matthew's! His lean at the end clinched his third-place spot and sent him on to state once again. Though the other boy cried and cried, he did go on to state in the 100, taking third place right in front of Matthew! Shocker, huh!!! Oh my goodness, my heart pounds even now as I remember what happened.

All I can say is that it is a darn good thing I train hard and eat right because I almost had heart failure as the night unfolded. Those of you who have children, or plan to in the future, please take care of yourself. If you don't, times like these might just kill you!

I included this story in a chapter on character because the word *character* means "an account of the Christ-like qualities or peculiarities of a person or thing." In essence, our character is formed by an account of our actions. Our actions determine the quality of character in each of us. Matthew's character as revealed by the account of his actions at this track meet has little to do with whether or not he won his race. Rather, his character is revealed by the Christ-like actions he displayed from beginning to end.

As you learned in the TAP principle and "I Am" declaration, you must control or take captive your thoughts and make them obedient to Christ. You must stay in spiritual alignment with God, beginning with what and how you think, the attitude that comes with it, and the performance or actions that follow. How well you learn to do this is what shapes your character. If you read the story again, you will see that Matthew's thoughts, attitude, and performance were in alignment with God.

How many of us would rather run the race again and lose than win with a coin-toss and go to state? It was late and already past his bedtime, and yet he chose to *earn* his way to state rather than leave it to the chance. When Matthew saw how upset the boy was when he found out he had to run again, he even encouraged the other boy by saying, "You can do this! You have a good chance and might even beat me!" The other boy wouldn't even look at Matthew. Instead, he cried because he didn't want to run again. Matthew actually served and blessed his opponent by encouraging him and even let him choose the lane. Remember the scripture where Jesus tells us to love our enemies and to bless those who persecute us? This is what it looks like. No, the boy wasn't his enemy per se. But so many times in this world an opponent is seen as an enemy! Whether or not Matthew won the race, he was already a winner. The other boy's father couldn't believe it when Matthew gave his son the choice of lanes.

Here is the catch. Though Matthew appeared confident and very secure, his body was nervous and under pressure. He could feel his adrenaline kick in and even experienced fear. But despite his fear, he found his courage. He took captive his thoughts of possible defeat, his attitude of fear, and gave them to God. He knew that God would give him what he needed when he needed it, and this calmed his body down before the race. Thus he not only conquered his own fear, but tried helping his opponent conquer his fear. Matthew wanted his opponent at his best so they would have an awesome race. Talk about character.

Everything you do to practice putting your thoughts, attitudes, and performances in alignment with God shapes your character. Your health and fitness is a huge part of what shapes your character. Every time you mentally choose the action of exercise, despite how you may or may not feel, you shape your character. Every time you are tired but keep your commitment to train anyway, you shape your character. Every time you choose healthy food when something unhealthy is staring you in the face, you shape your character. Every time you choose to persevere when you don't feel like it, you shape your character. Choosing to run the race even when you are tired is what shapes your character. Every time you take captive your defeating thoughts and attitudes and change them into positive, life-affirming thoughts and attitudes, you shape your character.

Others always see character in your actions but you alone experience it first in your thoughts and attitude. Good character always has all three components of the TAP principle working together, whether good, bad, or indifferent. The kind of character you want is Christ-like.

How many of us could say that we lovingly encourage the very opponents who are out to beat us? How many of us act as Matthew did in my story? Well, only you know the answer to these questions. But, of course, even Matthew at times makes the wrong choices. I know I certainly do. But as we as a family practice the principles of TAP and the "I Am" on a daily basis, the amount of good character choices increases and our fleshly ways of stinkin' thinkin' dwindle away. Jesus came to heal the sick, and that means *all of us*. Only Jesus in His perfection had unblemished character. But as we increase our love affair with Him, He will lead us into a life in which His character becomes our own. And when we fall short, He will be there to cover us, love us, and forgive us. After all, just as with obedience, our Christ-like character comes *from* our love affair with Christ. It doesn't get us *to* Him! It is simply a reflection of our complete surrender to His will in our lives.

Watch as God builds your character through the healthy choices you make. Watch as worldly control and addictions dwindle away as you focus on building your Christ-like character. Be good to yourself and make choices out of the overflow of love that only God can give you.

For Reflection:

What does the statement "our Christ-like character comes *from* our love affair with Christ. It doesn't get us *to* Him!" mean to you?

_____

_____

What healthy choices are you making that God can use to build your character?

_____

_____

BUILDING RELATIONSHIPS

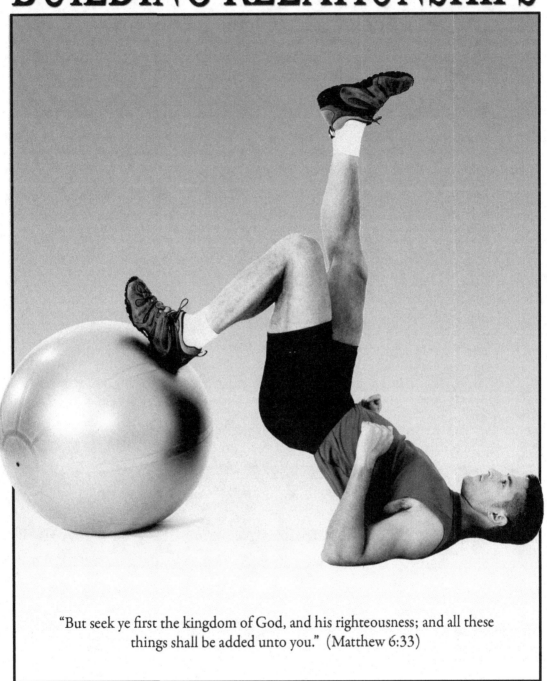

"But seek ye first the kingdom of God, and his righteousness; and all these things shall be added unto you." (Matthew 6:33)

WEEK TEN

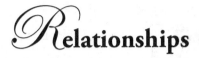

Relationships

"Lining up your priorities with God"

As you learn to prioritize your time and energy, understand the reason you even have an order of things so you can build, cultivate, nurture, and cherish the relationships in your life. You don't follow an order because some legalistic command orders you to submit or be subject to the wrath of God. You follow an order because you are here on this earth to be in beautiful, flourishing relationships. God wants to see His love made manifest in your life by how you treat yourself and others with love and kindness.

Whenever your priorities and time commitments are out of balance in any way, it will affect your relationships—all of them, including the one you have with yourself. Does your household resemble a boarding house or dormitory whose residents basically eat and sleep there but have little or no interaction with each other? Does your family have so much going on that it is difficult to connect with each other on any level? Do you sometimes feel as though you are simply a shuttle service instead of a family? Do any of these questions ring a bell? Yes, we are busy people, but too many "tasky" things keep us from being connected to each other. Taking inventory of where your priorities are is vital as you focus on your relationships.

So where do relationships start? Review the *Tree of Life* on the following page so you can see the order of things. It goes like this; God, self/health, family, career, and then ministry. The same goes with your relationships. This is so important that you may wonder why I didn't put it in the front of the book and journal. Listen carefully. How can you understand priorities and an order of things if you do not first understand who you are, your value, where it comes from, and why and where your old patterns of behavior need to change? How can you possibly look at your schedule and your relationships with a mindset of positive change with your old eyes, old ears, and old ways? Over the past 10–11 weeks, you have been changing from the inside out, taking captive your thoughts and attitude, losing weight, and taking care of yourself. You are in a better place, and with that in mind let's dive into the beauty of "priorities" and how they affect relationships.

The following diagram shows you the tree of life.

Tree of Life

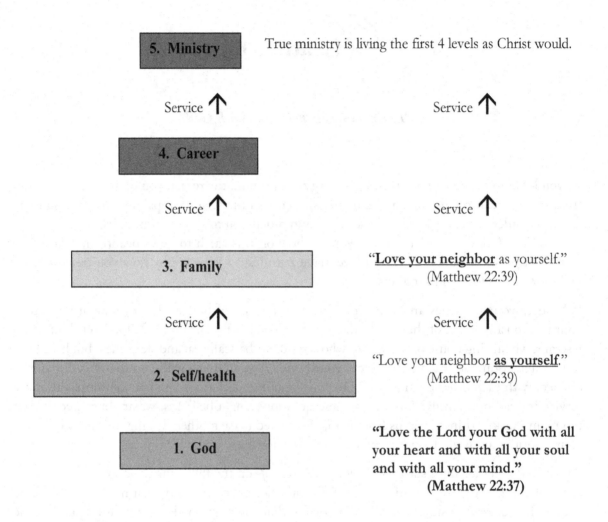

The first two levels of the Tree of Life set the foundation in your life so you can serve the way God has called you to serve: effectively, abundantly, and powerfully! **"Love the Lord your God with all your heart and with all your soul and with all your mind"** and **"Love your neighbor AS YOURSELF."**

1. Your relationship with God

Your first and most important relationship is the one you have with God, with Christ, and/or the Holy Trinity (Father, Son, and Holy Spirit). Remember the first of the two great commandments: **"Love the Lord your God with all your heart and with all your soul and with all your mind"** (Matthew 22:37). Why would God say this? Why would He give this as a command? It is because He loves you and wants a relationship with you, with each and every one of us. You are His precious son or daughter and He is always in pursuit of your heart, soul, mind, and strength. The only way to cultivate this relationship is by being in communion with Him constantly—all day, every day—to crave your moment-by-moment love affair with Jesus. It is the most amazing, mind-blowing, incredible relationship you will ever have. Over and over God tells you that He craves this intimacy with you.

2. Your relationship with yourself

Many of you have grown up hearing the words *God, family,* and *career.* But where do *you* fit into this picture? Is "self" important? Are *you* important? The answer is YES. Ultimately your life is about God, not you, but how can you truly serve and love others if you do not first love yourself? The second great commandment says, "Love your neighbor as yourself." You are to have a relationship with and love God as the greatest commandment, yes, but you are commanded also to love yourself in Matthew 22:37. This love of self is what enables you to have a relationship with and love others.

You cultivate and nurture family, career, and ministry relationships as the result of God's love and gifts being poured into your heart and of *your* owning the truth about who God has created you to be.

Your body is perhaps God's most basic gift to you. Your health is perhaps your most basic gift to God. Your overall health is about love. How you live each moment with love is manifested into relationship. There is physical health, mental health, emotional health, and spiritual health, all of which directly affect each other and are based on relationship.

Throughout *Courage to Change* you have been learning that *you* matter, that your health matters, that God cares about *you!*

Who are you? What gives you passion? What foods do you like? Do you like the ocean or do you like the mountains? What is your favorite color? Though life is about God, not you, He created you to be different from any other person on the planet, with unique gifts and special likes and dislikes. One way to strengthen your relationship with God is to learn all you can about how He made you and then to love yourself as His wonderful, beautiful creation. You then honor the love you have for yourself by taking care of the wonderful creation God made in you. He gave you your very own mind to think with. He gave you your very own heart to give and receive love with. And He gave you your very own beautiful body to be a good steward over.

Your love for yourself is still about God and not about you. As you love yourself, you are living in gratitude and thankfulness to God for how He made you. God says you were wonderfully and fearfully made, but how do you know this unless you get to know and love yourself through God's eyes? When you put that love into action, then you are preserving the beauty of what God has made in you. Even your body is to be used for honoring Him and ultimately for serving others.

In the airline industry, they teach you to put the oxygen mask on yourself first, then on your kids. Why? To be selfish? No! Because you aren't going to be any good to your children if you pass out and die. Which is better—saving five people and then suffocating, or putting the oxygen mask on yourself first, then saving 50 people, and going on to live because you could breathe? Your health is the greatest example of this scenario. I wish my father were around to see his grandchildren. But because he never took care of himself, he died of a massive heart attack at the age of 61. My biological father didn't raise me, but he is not here to see his grandchildren, either. He didn't take care of himself and died of a heart attack at the age of 39. Both of my dads mattered to me, and they especially mattered to God. My relationship with them was cut short because they had no idea who they were and the importance of "self."

Again, I am not talking about the selfish, prideful self here, but the self that God wants us to love in the "as yourself" part of the second greatest commandment, "Love your neighbor **as yourself**" (Matthew 22:39).

You see, you have a relationship with yourself! It is your responsibility to make yourself a priority in your life, to schedule things in your life that pertain just to you. Your health is about putting on your oxygen mask first so that you can then help others more effectively. Along with a health regimen, schedule relaxation time, fun time, and prayer time into your weeks. They don't have to be long periods either. I know you are all busy. I know I am. But you absolutely need time for yourself, to get to know yourself, to build your relationship with yourself. Otherwise, you become a walking zombie full of stress and disarray.

Imagine for a moment that the relationship between you and God and you and "you" is the foundation of a building or house. What is the purpose of a foundation? A foundation's purpose is to support whatever is erected on top of it. But what makes a foundation strong? Did you know that concrete by itself is crumbly and breaks very easily? But when you add sand and steal bars called rebar to the concrete it becomes strong enough to support massive 200 story skyscrapers and interstates you can drive on. Think of God as the sand and rebar that strengthens and reinforces the concrete (you) so the two of you can support what you build together…beautiful relationships! The building or house the two of you build together represents your family, friends, businesses, and ministries. **That is why every single relationship beyond this point is about serving.**

3. Your relationships with your family

After you cultivate a relationship with God and yourself, your family comes next. Bruce Wilkerson put it this way, "The home is the single greatest arena on earth to change a life for God." The home is the most vulnerable, yet intimate, place on earth. It is where people spend the most time together and where we see the best of the best and the worst of the worst in people. Home is where the good, the bad, and the ugly happen. It is the hardest yet most rewarding part of our relationships because it takes an awful lot of humility, trust, patience, tolerance, kindness, and emotional investment. *Courage to Change* has hopefully equipped you with tools to know how to change your family legacy from negative to positive, from unhealthy to healthy. But as you continue to practice the principles in *Courage to Change*, you need to be mindful of the order that God has established in your family.

The order is husband, wife, then kids. Notice that mother- or father-in-law isn't present. It says in Genesis 2:24, **"A man will leave his father and mother and be united to his wife, and they will become one flesh."** Once you are married, your parents are to stay out of the way. You must break free. Moms and dads, if your kids are married, don't think you have the same relationship you did when they were single. You are no longer a part of their immediate family. Though you are still instrumental in their life, you now come after their spouses and children.

God is very clear in His word about who is the head of the house. It's the wife, of course. OK, OK, so scripture says the husband is the head of the house and his wife is to submit to him. **"Wives, submit to your husbands as to the Lord. For the husband is the head of the wife as Christ** is the head of the church, his body, of which he is the Savior. Now as the church submits to Christ, so also wives should submit to their husbands in everything" (Ephesians 5:22-24). Now don't panic, ladies, you have the power. This is actually a beautiful principle. **Here is the clincher, ladies: It is up to you to choose a man worthy of submitting to!**

A man's serving as the head of the house simply means that he has the greatest responsibility to be a spiritual covering for his family. He is supposed to be a rock, a godly man whose purpose is to lift up each member of his family. A man is commanded to love his wife as Christ loved His church and died for it.

> **"Husbands, love your wives, just as Christ loved the church and gave himself up for her to make her holy, cleansing her by the washing with water through the word, and to present her to himself as a radiant church, without stain or wrinkle or any other blemish, but holy and blameless. In this same way, husbands ought to love their wives as their own bodies. He who loves his wife loves himself."** (Ephesians 5:25–28)

Sounds pretty good, doesn't it, ladies? It is up to you to have enough confidence and self-worth that the only man worth your time is one who knows and is completely sold out to Jesus Christ, one who will die for you, one who will present you to Him as a radiant church. He won't dominate you and keep you from being your best. He will help *guide* you into being *your* best. He will listen to your wisdom and guidance but will take everything to the Lord out of humility and submission. **He isn't the all powerful leader or dictator but is the greatest servant among the family. After all, he is supposed to be an example of Christ. Jesus came not to rule, but to serve!**

As I stated in the "Legalism" section of *Courage to Change*, I once worked with a very legalistic man. I once overheard him arguing with a client over his role in marriage. He was about to get married, and evidently it came up in the conversation as he and the client were in the gym training. My partner refused to listen to the man share his heart about the importance of listening to his wife and realizing that she was there to minister to and hold him accountable. The client told him that the reason his own marriage had ended in a bitter divorce was because he had never listened to his ex-wife. He had verbally abused her and kept her in her place as "less than." My partner said over and over, "I will be the head of the house and she will do what I say! That is scriptural and that is final." I wanted to call his poor fiancée and tell her to run as fast as she could. Men, if you think that being the head of the house means being a dictator and use your spiritual authority to abuse and manipulate your wife or girlfriend, you are out of the will of God and it needs to stop! What you need is a swift kick in the fanny and a smack upside your head. Having said all that, Ladies, please don't expect your husband to be Jesus himself. Even the most godly of men are going to make mistakes. I know I certainly do.

I don't know a single woman who doesn't like to feel safe. Yes, a woman can live without a man and can do just as well, but there is a spiritual covering and protection from a godly man that comes with marriage. It is in a man's nature to protect. Even if a woman makes 10 times the money of her husband, the husband will still feel the pressure to provide for his family because it is in his nature to protect and provide. So, ladies, submit to your husbands out of love and let your husbands cover you. Men, step up to the plate and be the men of God your families deserve. Lead with love and gentleness and teach your children the ways of the Lord.

So where do the children fit in? How many families in this day and age are run by the children? Everything is about the kids. Kids this and kids that. The father and mother are the center of the house—not the children. If a family has this mixed up, the children will grow up not knowing what submission is all about. They learn how to submit to God from first revering and submitting to their parents. This doesn't mean that the children do not count or have a voice. It simply means that parents are the authority and are due respect and honor.

> **"Children, obey your parents in the Lord, for this is right. Honor your father and mother—which is the first commandment with a promise—that it may go well with you and that you may enjoy long life on the earth."** (Ephesians 6:1–3)

This scripture passage is very important. Silesia and I have seen over and over the legalistic repercussions of abusing Ephesians 6:1–3. It says in Ephesians 6:4, **"Fathers, do not exasperate your children; instead, bring them up in the training and instruction of the Lord."** If children are ignored or made to feel as though they are not important, it is wrong. I learn as much from my children as I do from anyone else. If I listen to them, I get a front-row seat to hear the Holy Spirit speaking through them. **"From the lips of children and infants you have ordained praise because of your enemies, to silence the foe and the avenger"** (Psalms 8:2). Don't let your children get so busy that they don't enjoy their childhood. They will simply grow up and not enjoy their adulthood either. Their lives will be filled with "stuff." Of course, you should always teach your children to strive for excellence, but there is a balance, and too much is too much.

Why would I be covering these things in a book on health and fitness? The reason is that there are only so many hours in a day. So many of you, myself included (in the past), have filled your days up with so much stuff that it is virtually impossible to start taking care of yourself. "I just don't have the time." "My kids just take up too much of my time." In setting your priorities of relationship-building you will find (make) the time to take care of yourself. Many of you need to reorganize and reprioritize your lives so that they follow the order that God has laid out. If you have no time to exercise or fix healthy food, then somewhere you are out of balance. It needs to change.

4. Your relationships with career

I believe that each person has not only a spiritual purpose but a "work purpose" as well. God will use your gifts to help navigate you into a career where you can honor Him with the talents and abilities He gave you. After all, the entire workforce is about relationship, about serving one another. Every single product, store, or service, is about doing one thing: serving others in some way. Some industries are good and some are bad.

Many clients throughout my career have changed jobs, started their own businesses, or even broken sales goals after beginning *Courage to Change*. The reason is that they tap into their passions, their purpose, and their greatness, all of which were given to them by God. Doing the actions necessary to be healthy sparks action in all areas of their lives.

So many people see themselves in a dead-end job and just can't seem to get motivated. Well, if you remember in Week 1 of *Courage to Change*, *motivation* in Hebrew means "God's energy." Building your relationship with God and getting to know yourself may stoke that fire in your current job or give you the desire to find a job more suited to your gifts. All in all, there is an order found in business, just as in everything else.

Your supervisor or boss is your authority at work. So many people rebel against their authority because they think that they are owed something from the company they work for. You cannot live this way. Romans states clearly that you are to submit yourself to the governing authorities. This means in business, government, and the church:

> **"Everyone must submit . . . to the governing authorities, for there is no authority except that which God has established. The authorities that exist have been established by God. Consequently, he who rebels against the authority is rebelling against what God has instituted, and those who do so will bring judgment on themselves. For rulers hold no terror for those who do right, but for those who do wrong. Do you want to be free from fear of the one in authority? Then do what is right and he will commend you. For he is God's servant to do you good. But if you do wrong, be afraid, for he does not bear the sword for nothing. He is God's servant, an agent of wrath to bring punishment on the wrongdoer. Therefore, it is necessary to submit to the authorities, not only because of possible punishment but also because of conscience. This is also why you pay taxes, for the authorities are God's servants, who give their full time to governing."** (Romans 13:1-6)

If you don't like your job, or your boss is a control freak, then get a different job—but as long as you are there, you need to do your job. Stop the grumbling and complaining and do not think that the company owes you anything because of your sweet presence. Either do your job or move on. **Here is the clincher: It is up to you to choose a job or career with supervisors worthy of submitting to!** *You* **have the power, not they.**

If submitting to the authority in your job means compromising your standards or subjecting your spirit to anger or control, then do what is right and either go higher up in the chain of command to be heard or find another job! When you go on a job interview, it is just as much your interview as it theirs. If they don't line up with your morals and the Holy Spirit puts up a red flag or sounds a siren, then move on and find something else. You need to know that *you have options! Yes, even in a hurting economy!*

How in the world are you going to find the energy to take care of yourself if you are in constant stress at work? And even if things are going well at work, take inventory. Do you put work before your family? Do you put work before your health? Do you say such things as, "I just don't have the time to take care of myself. I just have too much work to do." Well, who is in charge of your life—you or your work? If you need to make changes, make them, but don't let yourself get caught up in the mindset that there is nothing you can do about it or say such things as, "That's just the way life is." *No, sir!* That's *not* just the way life is. You take control of your life and make the necessary changes you need to be healthy.

5. Your relationships with ministry

Your relationships in ministry come after the previous four in terms of priority. I have seen people over and over submerge themselves in ministry and in the process neglect their health, career, family, and oddly enough even their relationship with God. How is this possible? Oftentimes, you get insecure in yourself, and instead of breaking that stranglehold, you reinforce it by focusing all of your energy on others. Sure, you are to serve others, but *not* at the expense of your own health and well-being. By not honoring the second great commandment of "loving your neighbor *as yourself*," you open yourself to a downward spiral of low self-esteem, feelings of unworthiness, and poor self-image. Remember, though, you know that God loves you and that He is where you get your value; the way you honor that love and value is by your loving actions of taking care of yourself inside and out.

Placing others before or above you does not mean totally ignoring your own needs and seeing yourself as lowly or *less than*. If you think very highly of yourself (in terms of accepting who you are in Christ) and love yourself and then put others before you, then God will better elevate them through your encouragement! Ministry is not only going out into the mission field, it is also lining up your priorities in the right order. Your whole life is a ministry. So please do not use ministry to hide behind poor health! Do not use it as an excuse to not take care of yourself. Realign and reprioritize your life so that it reflects the right order. Then you will not only work in or be involved in ministry but your entire life will be a ministry by the example you set.

Too often our spouses and children think that they come second to ministry and work. Though parents may verbally profess their love for their children, their actions may show otherwise. The same goes for the spouse. Our children and spouses need to know that they come before work and before ministry. They learn this by watching what we do, not by hearing what we say. Your *Life Application Journal* poses a number of questions to help you determine where you are. Whatever changes you need to make, make them, without guilt or shame. As God leads you to the areas you need to change, simply say, "I get to change."

Again, your health will not become a priority unless you reevaluate your priorities. As you learn how to do this, be aware of a behavior that we have all been guilty of from time to time—"compartmentalizing," which we will look at in the next section. Understanding compartmentalizing will give you an even better idea of how you have been prioritizing your time and your thought processes in the middle of it and how to change it.

For Reflection:

List the top 5 priorities in your life in order from most to least important (based on your actions not how you think they *should* be).

_____

_____

What changes (if any) do you need to make in order to align your priorities with the order revealed in God's word?

_____

_____

Compartmentalizing

"Forgetting about the many needs and demands of your body, mind, and Spirit while focusing on one thing at a time"

"I just don't have the time. I'm too tired at the end of the day. I just have too much going on right now. I am beautiful on the inside." These thoughts and ideas have made their way into the minds of millions of people. They are lies from the enemy and constantly hold you back by justifying your decision *not to act*. What behavioral mindset can you look at that may tell you why you think that way? One such mindset is compartmentalizing.

Compartmentalizing is forgetting about the many needs and demands of your body, mind, and spirit while focusing on one thing at a time. Many of you forget about your body as you go to work. Many of you have forgotten your relationship with God, your wife, and your friends as you go to work. When you go to church, you take your "church-self" with you. When you go to work, you take your "work-self" with you. When you go out with friends, you take your "partying-self" with you and forget about your spirit and body and the consequences of unhealthy choices. **Remember, every part of you goes with you wherever you go, and God is always there with you as well.** All parts of you coexist. Your body requires care and nourishment wherever you go—whether at work, on vacation, or out with friends. While at work, you may need to focus on your job, but you should always keep your awareness on the other equally important components of your life.

Your body is one of the main areas of neglect when you compartmentalize. As you take each part of you wherever you go and balance your life on the fulcrum of God, observe as He shows you how to be healthy regardless of your situation and busy schedule.

Solutions to Compartmentalizing as it pertains to your health

a. God goes with you everywhere you go. Be aware of His presence in you at all times and let Him lead you in every decision, every thought, every attitude, and every performance (TAP).

b. When you are busy with work and daily activities, it is hard to remember to eat when you need to, especially when you are first starting this program and making changes. If you work on a computer terminal, program your computer to remind you to eat every three hours throughout the day.

c. Many wrist watches can be programmed to beep every three hours to remind you to eat your next meal. Whether in the office, at home, or in outside sales, this is a great way to remind yourself to eat and take care of yourself.

d. Almost all cell phones now have a way for you to set multiple alarms (with memos) throughout the day, reminders to eat and exercise when it is time.

e. If you have an assistant or receptionist, have him or her remind you each day of the times to eat, just as you would be reminded of an important client meeting. But remember that the responsibility is *yours*. Hopefully your receptionist or assistant is on this program, too, so your whole office can do it as a team.

f. Plan for when you are weak. It isn't a matter of *if*, but *when*. When do you make bad choices nutritionally? When you are hungry. Prepare food in advance. Have low-fat protein bars available. Keep water bottles in your car and office.

g. Keep pictures of your family on your desk and in your wallet or purse. Call or text-message once in a while just to say, "I love you."

h. Eat breakfast and dinner as a family.

i. When out with friends, remember that God is with you. With Him you have a much greater chance of not compromising your health on all levels. That doesn't mean not having a cheeseburger once in a while. But without God, it is very difficult to be responsible to a committed goal, especially when you are out with friends who might not be working the program.

j. Remember that wherever you go, all of you goes, too! Stay true to the order found in this section and you will find your life a lot less stressful. Building relationships starts with God. Watch how your life changes. Just remember that *you* are important to God. The relationship you have with *you* and God lays the foundation for you to be able to love and serve others.

For Reflection:

In what areas of your life are you prone to compartmentalizing? For example, "When I'm at work, I neglect to…."

_____

_____

What are some specific actions you can take to de-compartmentalize?

_____

_____

Law of First Fruits

"Willingly and lovingly giving away at least the first 10% of God's gifts you want more of in return"

The law of first fruits is also about your relationships and lining your priorities up with God. Your desire to reap a bountiful harvest in every area of your life is founded on giving. Every form of giving is about relationship—with God, yourself, and others. Throughout the scriptures we are told that it is better to give than to receive, that those who give reap a bountiful harvest. The law of first fruits is a willing and loving giving away of at least the first 10% of God's gifts you want more of in return. The interesting part of the law of first fruits is that it holds true to every area of life, including your health.

Listen carefully! Isn't it interesting that to receive more physical energy, you must first be willing to give away or expend energy in the form of exercise? Isn't it interesting that to lose weight, you must burn more calories than you consume, or, put another way, that you must give away more calories than you take in or receive? It is the same with love, money, patience, forgiveness, and any of the other gifts from God that you want more of in return.

This is why exercise is a form of worship as you offer your body as a living sacrifice, holy and pleasing to God. As you do your part by giving away your physical energy, God does His part by giving you more energy than you started with.

> **"'Bring the whole tithe into the storehouse, that there may be food in my house. Test me in this,' says the LORD Almighty, 'and see if I will not throw open the floodgates of heaven and pour out so much blessing that you will not have room enough for it. I will prevent pests from devouring your crops, and the vines in your fields will not cast their fruit,' says the LORD Almighty."** (Malachi 3:10–11)

Though God is speaking about a bountiful harvest of finances here, the tithe and first portion, or 10%, of the tithe is a law that extends into every area of your life. The more you give, the more you receive. When you hoard money, it controls you. What happens when you hoard energy in the form of calories? You get out of shape, obese, sluggish, and sickly. When you don't expend or give away those calories, they are stored up and are not being used for you.

Remember: **To receive more physical energy, you must first be willing to give it away.** The more you live by this principle, the greater abundance God will give you in each area of your life.

In addition to the example I just gave regarding physical energy, tithing is a beautiful way to honor God. First of all, the word *tithe* actually means 10, and God asks us to tithe this amount off the top of our financial increase (Malachi 3:10–11). God actually asks us to test Him on this! Without going into a long, in-depth study of tithing, I will share with you a couple of personal stories of God's faithfulness as a result of my obedience in tithing.

Doubling Down ... and Receiving God's Blessing

Earlier in my career in Denver, I tithed $20 per week when I went to church because that was what I grew up thinking my father tithed. I would later find out that he had tithed well above and beyond the Sunday offering of $20. But since that is what I saw, that is what I did. The longer I worked in Denver, the more I learned how to build my business into a flourishing practice. As I became more educated and designed the original version of *Courage to Change*, I also learned how to market myself. My business practically doubled overnight. Months at a time I would get two or three new clients every week. But after a while, all of the sudden it stopped. Over a period of three weeks I didn't receive so much as one phone call from someone new. Though I was doing quite well, this drought of calls made me nervous. I remember sitting down on the gliding rocker in my apartment one Sunday morning before church and wondering what was going on. It didn't make sense.

As I sat and pondered my circumstances, I began to pray. At that time I didn't know Jesus on an intimate level. I believed in Him but was unaware of the intimate relationship He so deeply wanted with me. I did pray, however. After a while a thought came to my mind. Here my business was doing better than ever before and was making twice as much money as before, yet I was still tithing just $20 per week. I became excited to get to church so I could give more! That morning I doubled my tithe. Instead of giving $20, I gave $40. At that point I didn't know that *tithe* meant 10%, and I still wasn't tithing 10%. I just knew that I needed to give more because I was making more.

So off to church I went and smiled as I dropped my tithe into the basket as it went by. I didn't do it with grumbling or because I felt I had to. I did it because of how thankful I was that my business was doing so well. I went about my day and went to sleep that night feeling good. I had no idea what I would wake up to.

I went to work the next morning at my usual time of 5:30 and checked my voice mail to see if any of my clients had canceled that morning. But what do you think I heard? Not only had no clients canceled, but I had voice mails from three new prospective clients. I hadn't received a single phone call in three weeks, and the very day after I increased my tithe, they were there. It was so weird and kind of freaky. My faith was definitely increased that day. Over and over God has delivered His promise in this way.

Learning to Rely on God's Provision

The next experience has unfolded over time. At the time I began tithing more, it was also the time I felt God pursuing me, wanting me to know that there was something amazing He wanted to show me about Himself. Without going into my whole story, it was a three-to-four-year transformation during which I went from being blind to seeing very clearly. I left Denver to move to Dallas because I was miserable. Something was gnawing at me, and that *something* was God wanting to show me the intimacy He wanted with me. He wanted me to experience the intimate love affair with Jesus. Next thing I knew, all hell had broken loose in my life. I dropped everything and went on the most amazing, mind-blowing journey with God I had ever experienced.

About halfway through this amazing transformation, I was living with a young couple in Pantego, Texas. They owned a health facility and offered me a place to stay as I got my feet back on the ground. I was making mere pennies and could barely pay for dog food for my dog, Faith. At this time God was teaching me so many different things. I was learning how to receive from people and how to rely on God's provisions. I was also learning the difference between confidence and arrogance. I was driving a black turbo diesel Excursion with oversized tires. Boy, was it cool. OK, single guy, no family, no house…who drives a bus! The huge Excursion represented the pride in my right pinky toe. But God was patient with me as he showed me. . . *me!*

My love for God and the intimacy I experienced grew daily. It was amazing. I was sold. I wanted to honor Him with all of me and continually asked Him to mold me and further transform me into His image. Did I mention that I was leasing the Excursion at $600 per month? It was something I didn't even own. *Oh my!* It was eating my lunch financially. I could barely afford to make the payments and couldn't afford the insurance. In fact, I was two months behind when I went to God for some answers. I wanted to be a good steward over my commitment to my lease. But what I found was that I couldn't be a good steward over taking care of *me* by keeping the Excursion. It was me or the bus! What made me feel even worse was that I couldn't afford to tithe my 10% to the church because it was all tied up with the Excursion. This experience also showed me my future. Was I willing to do what I needed to do to provide for my future family?

I sought some counsel and made a decision that changed my life. It was more important to me to tithe my 10% than to keep my Excursion, so I voluntarily turned it in. My love for God had finally exceeded my pride. My arrogance was replaced with humility and God's love. For the next six months, I rode my bike 10–20 miles per day to and from work. Whether it rained or was 105 degrees, I rode. I still designed programs for people and rode my bike another 10 miles to Kinko's to have them printed up. But while I rode, I knew that God was with me, and I felt such a peace that I was now able to tithe my 10%. I even rode my bike to church with dress clothes on and a Bible under my arm. Nothing could keep me from going. It was then that I started to get my feet back on the ground. After that, I still had many obstacles to conquer as God continued changing my heart and mind. He delivered me from so many things. My whole story is a true testament of the amazing power and grace that comes in a relationship with Jesus.

Fast forward three years. I now have a wonderful wife, two kids, and a house and continue to tithe over 10% of our income. Because I started over and did it God's way, we as a family are also completely debt-free. He is an awesome God.

Give out of the love you have in your heart. Share with your kids what you give, how much you give, and where it goes. It wasn't until three years after my father's death that I found out how much he had given through tithing and charitable contributions. I had no idea how much he had done. So talk to your children and share with them what you do.

As you long to know Christ more intimately, your love will increase and so will your willingness to give. Believe in His provisions for you. He did it for me and He will do it for you.

For Reflection:

Are there some areas of your life—finances, gifts, talents, etc.—in which you have been holding back or holding out on God?

_____

_____

What can you do right now to "double down" and give more of your first fruits?

_____

_____

A CALL TO ACTION

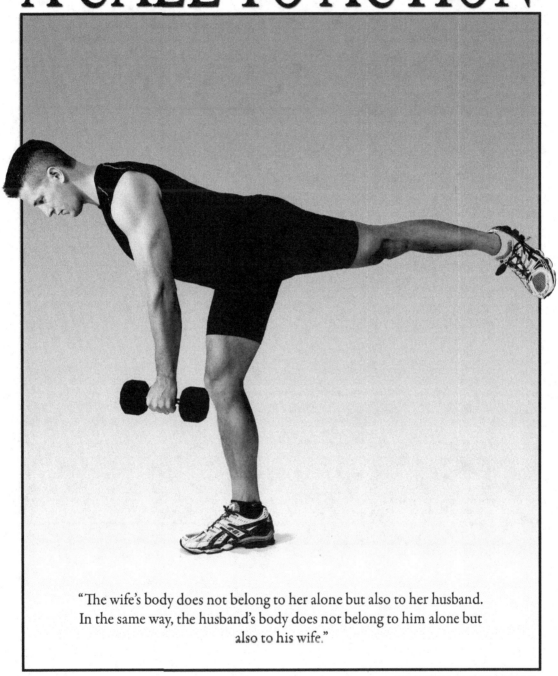

"The wife's body does not belong to her alone but also to her husband. In the same way, the husband's body does not belong to him alone but also to his wife."

WEEK ELEVEN

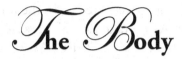The Body

"Just as each of us has one body with many members, and these members do not all have the same function, so in Christ we who are many form one body, and each member belongs to all the others." (Romans 12:4–5)

As you answer the call to action, consider your gifts and the unique part you play in the body of Christ. Did you know that you were created different from any other person on earth? Did you know that even the way you experience God is different from everyone else? Why or how? You ask. Because He made you as a unique and precious work of art and gave you special gifts that drive you and make you *you*. And God made you not only physically different but *spiritually* different as well. The more you get to know yourself and learn about how God wired you, the better you will be at setting, reaching, and surpassing your goals because you will realize that God—the Tailor—designed you for excellence in every area of your life. Let's start with your body and go from there.

Your body is an engineering marvel. *You* are an engineering marvel. God designed your body to be strong and fight off disease, but because we live in a "fallen" world because of sin, your body is also weak and vulnerable and must be treated with care. Your body can persevere when called upon to perform but it can break down when it becomes too tired. Consider this, the human body is the only thing God created in the whole universe that actually gets stronger, shinier, and healthier the more you use it. Contrast this with a brand-new baseball. Soon it has a grass stain on it. It then turns brown from water and dirt. The bat takes its toll and before long the baseball begins to lose its shape. It gets scuffed and torn as it slams into fences and breaks the neighbor's windows. The only way to keep it white and in "brand-new condition" is to never use it and keep it in an airtight case. But not you, not your body. Your bruises heal. The cut you get reaching through the neighbor's broken window to retrieve that errant baseball closes up and heals itself. The more you run, leap, prance, sweat, and use your muscles, the stronger you get and the more vitality you acquire. The more you use your lungs, the stronger they get. The faster your heart beats during physical exertion, the slower yet more powerful it beats when you are at rest. Your bones and muscles become stronger as you add resistance to your workouts, and your muscles become more flexible as you stretch them. Your senses become heightened and your body more relaxed and de-stressed as you use your body the way it was designed. But if you sit and do nothing, your body breaks down. God is so amazing.

Only as Strong as the Weakest Link

God reveals His very nature to us as we take care of ourselves. Chances are, you have never truly experienced this phenomenon. All of us were created in the image of God, and that image is no still portrait. It is an action film. As we take care of ourselves, we learn how God designed us individually and corporately as "the body of Christ." As we love ourselves and our individual bodies with action, we learn how we are also integral parts of a much larger body. Each link in a chain has its own function, but that function is limited unless the link is connected to the others to form the whole chain. We must realize that if even one link in a chain is rusty and not oiled, it will eventually affect the entire chain. Sooner or later the chain will break because of that neglected link. We as the church body, the body of Jesus Christ, must see ourselves as a link in a chain, a chain of love. Each of us must do our part in keeping physically strong and oiled individually, and all of us together must keep our "body" as a unit in good shape. Isn't it the chain that drives the bike forward as the pedals go round and round? As you heal, I heal. As I heal, you heal because we are connected.

Are we not all called as a church body to move together, as a unit, while being strong individually? Even the Bible compares your body and how it works with "the body of Christ." How often have you seen people go into a gym and sit on machines that work only one specific muscle, while the rest of the body is inactive and asleep? My other books will explain this in more detail, but what good is an individual muscle if it doesn't know how to work as part of a whole unit? It is like having strong, well-oiled chain links that are not joined together. Collectively they cannot perform the way they need to perform. Later, you will learn about the concept of training the muscles of your body individually and as a unit simultaneously by performing functional movements, because the entire body must move to accomplish its goal. Isn't it just like God to show us this spiritual principle with our physical body?

> "For we were all baptized by one Spirit into one body—whether Jews or Greeks, slave or free—and we were all given the one Spirit to drink. Now the body is not made up of one part but of many. If the foot should say, 'Because I am not a hand, I do not belong to the body,' it would not for that reason cease to be part of the body. And if the ear should say, 'Because I am not an eye, I do not belong to the body,' it would not for that reason cease to be part of the body. If the whole body were an eye, where would the sense of hearing be? If the whole body were an ear, where would the sense of smell be? But in fact God has arranged the parts in the body, every one of them, just as he wanted them to be. If they were all one part, where would the body be? As it is, there are many parts, but one body. The eye cannot say to the hand, 'I don't need you!' And the head cannot say to the feet, 'I don't need you!' On the contrary, those parts of the body that seem to be weaker are indispensable, and the parts that we think are less honorable, we treat with special honor. And the parts that are unpresentable are treated with special modesty, while our presentable parts need no special treatment. But God has combined the members of the body and has given greater honor to the parts that lacked it, so that there should be no division in the body, but that its parts should have equal concern for each other. If one part suffers, every part suffers with

it; if one part is honored, every part rejoices with it. Now you are the body of Christ, and each one of you is a part of it." (1 Corinthians 12:13–27)

If I cut my finger, my whole body feels the pain and knows it is injured. If my heart stops beating, my entire body dies because no oxygen-rich blood is being pumped through the veins and arteries. **"If one part suffers, every part suffers with it; if one part is honored, every part rejoices with it."** A tiny cut on the pinky finger can eventually cause a whole 200-pound body to die. So remember that you are just as much a part of the body of Christ as the next person. You are just as important as your pastor or priest, brother or neighbor, and it is time you started acting accordingly. If you are unhealthy, if you do not take care of yourself, and if you are taking tons of pills and medications because of your inactive lifestyle, you are not only hurting yourself but the entire body of Christ. Ouch! That hurts doesn't it? Especially in the church, 20% of the people do 80% of the work. If this is you, you will get burned out and run down if you don't take of yourself.

You matter! You *are* important! Without you, the body doesn't function as it should. So the question is not whether or not you are a part of the body of Christ, but whether or not you are fulfilling your function within it. A muscle that is not used leads to overuse and overcompensation injuries for the other parts of the body that must do all the work. Are you the eye that sees or the ear that hears? Or maybe you are a tendon that holds two bones together in the rotator cuff of the church body. Maybe you are part of the hand that greets people with loving hugs and handshakes. Maybe you are a crucial part of the mitral valve in the heart which regulates blood flow into the body. Whatever your function is, it requires action, participation, strength, health, and endurance. So engage! Activate yourself and serve your function with action.

The Battle is On

You are fighting a very real war. You are fighting the war on disease, infirmity, sickness, and depression, most of which are brought on by complacency, laziness, and a general lack of action. So take the offensive! Take care of your body with good nutrition and exercise in a healthy way and watch as you become a "stronger, better functioning" member of the most important body ever—the body of Christ. After all, He sacrificed His body for you. Don't you think it's time you did the same for Him?

Cure for Yearning: Knowing Who You Are

You are here because you yearn for something. You may or may not be happy and joyful, but you sense that something is missing, something that you just can't quite put your finger on. You've tried weight-loss products before. You've tried working out. You've tried Bible study groups, reading books, writing poetry, spending more time with your spouse and children, and submerging yourself in your work. So why is there still that empty spot inside of you that cannot be filled up? Why do you feel there is more, as though there is something you are missing out on? Why do you so often fall short on the things you need to do for yourself and others—such as taking care of yourself with action?

So many Christ-followers don't know who they truly are, and so they fall short of doing what they need to do because they are unmotivated, uninspired, and unfulfilled. Before you can do anything for yourself, anything for others, or for God, you first must learn how to "*be*" you. So who are you? Are you a dentist, a baseball player, or a fisherman? Maybe you are a husband, a wife, a brother, or a real estate agent. Maybe you are a sanitation engineer, a good friend, a listener, or a singer. Maybe you are a combination of these things—and more—and are good at all or none of them. Maybe you have been very successful in some pursuits and failed miserably in others. So which of these says who you are? Which of these tells you your value as a man or woman?

None of them! They can't because these are things you "do," not who you are! Though we are all on a journey to find ourselves through God's leadership, we oftentimes place value on things we do, or don't do, while on that journey. Listen to me carefully and take heart as I ask you this first question. *What makes you think it is up to you to place value on your life?* You can't! Because all you can base it on is what you do, or don't do, in the eyes of God. If you are the one who places value on your life, what happens when you disobey, fail, or fall short of what God expects of you? Does your value lessen? Does your value decrease? As I sit here smiling at what you are about to learn, I wish I could see your face when you hear these next words.

You are not the one who dictates where your value lies and you never will be! God tells you how valuable you are. You are *this* valuable: **"For God so loved the world (YOU) that he gave His one and only Son, that whoever believes in Him shall not perish but have eternal life"** (John 3:16). But wait, there is more! How can that be possible? What could add to Jesus' dying on the cross and releasing us from sin? The answer is found in His resurrection. Get excited because you are about to discover your true value.

Jesus Christ knew only one thing—that He was His father's son. He knew nothing else. Only when He was secure in and ready as His father's son, did He "do" the things His father asked of Him. All He knew how to "be" was His father's son. He didn't try to "be" anything else. I'll say it again, *He was His father's son and that was all He knew how to be.* The things He did resulted directly from His knowing who He was. *You* must first "know that you know" who you are before you *do* anything for yourself or others. You are a son or daughter of the most high God and a member of His "royal family" as you welcome Him into your heart. Who else do you need to be but a son or daughter of your Father in heaven? Who else would you want to be? You can't change who you are, either. Jesus says it isn't you who chooses Him, but *He* who chooses you. Only when you accept who you *are* as a living, breathing son or daughter of God will you find peace in the things you *do* in your life. Once you realize who you are, you will learn that your Father in heaven has equipped you with everything you need to spread love to and receive love from others in the form of action. The reason you cannot determine your value or your worth is because you cannot give to yourself what God gives you through the Holy Spirit.

You are...A Beautiful Child of God

First of all, you are a beautiful child of God. I can tell you that you have been given gifts, amazing spiritual gifts, gifts of the Spirit. **Why? Because God loves you. You are His precious son or daughter. Take a moment to let this sink in before you continue reading.**

Before we learn how this happened, I will share one thing I have learned about gifts. Once we know what they are, they create a road map and tell us where we have been, where we are, and where we are going. Sure, we can recognize many talents, but certain ones *drive* us. Once I made the distinction between my talents and abilities in the things I did as a man and my gifts from God, my life made much more sense. As I learned about gifts and how God gave them to me, I could see how God was present in my life and worked through my gifts even before I truly knew Him. I was so amazed to learn of His awesome presence in my life even before I understood the concept of relationship and my love affair with Him. I now know why I have gone in the directions I have, faced the struggles I have gone through, and why sin appeared in my life where it did. I share these thoughts with you because I know you are on a lifelong journey of self-discovery and have possibly felt something missing in your life for a very long time. Once you learn your value as a man or woman you will have the motivation to "do" anything. You will find the drive and courage to build a business, lose weight, get in shape, spend more time with your spouse and children, and live each moment with enthusiasm. **What gives you that drive is knowing that no matter what you do, how well you succeed, or how miserably you fail, your value remains unblemished and purified through the blood of Jesus.**

I know you are excited. So am I! The next question is, "How" did this happen? How did you receive gifts from the Holy Spirit? Here's what happened. The Spirit of Jesus was released into your heart (as the Holy Spirit) when you made the decision to have a love affair with Him.

> **"God sent the Spirit of His Son into our hearts, the Spirit who calls out, 'Abba, Father.'"** (Galatians 4:6)

> **"Now the Lord is the Spirit, and where the Spirit of the Lord is, there is freedom. And we, who with unveiled faces all reflect the Lord's glory, are being transformed into his likeness with ever-increasing glory, which comes from the Lord, who is the Spirit."** (2 Corinthians 3:17–18)

The deeper your love affair with Christ and the more you explore your individual gifts, the more you understand that every person has been given gifts through the Holy Spirit who dwells inside of every believer. And that means *you!* In Romans 12:6–8, we are told, "**We have different gifts, according to the grace given us. If a man's gift is prophesying, let him use it in proportion to his faith. If it is serving, let him serve; if it is teaching, let him teach; if it is encouraging, let him encourage; if it is contributing to the needs of others, let him give generously; if it is leadership, let him govern diligently; if it is showing mercy, let him do it cheerfully.**" The gifts listed here in Romans are the gifts that drive all the others. They are the motivators we all have that lead into our other gifts. And though each one of us has every one of these gifts to some degree, we have one primary gift that drives us more than the others. My primary motivator is the gift of encouraging, with leadership coming in a very strong second. Why have I been in a position in my career that allows me to encourage and inspire people? Because I absolutely love it, and it is such a natural part of who I am. Why is my goal so strong that most of what I want to do with my life is bring out the best in people, to expose the power of God in each of you? It is because the primary gift that drives me is the gift of encouraging. Even as a young boy I loved encouraging people. My faith put into action is what manifests or nurtures these gifts. In essence God increases my desire for obedience and my ability to use my gifts as I display the intensity of my deep love for Him. So where are you?

What is Your Primary Gift?

My question is which primary motivator gift do you have? Yes, you have all the others, but there is one that drives you more than the others. It isn't something you appoint yourself. It is something the Holy Spirit reveals to you through prayer and obedience. It is evident in your fruit.

Understanding the unique gifts the Holy Spirit gives us helps us understand why we are told in Romans 12:4–5, **"Just as each of us has one body with many members, and these members do not all have the same function, so in Christ we who are many form one body, and each member belongs to all the others."** This is beautiful. We need each other and are commanded to love each other as Jesus loves us. As we learned earlier, we must love others as ourselves because we are part of one body in Christ. No one person has all the gifts working perfectly. That is why we are called to come together and work together in love so that we can build up the body of Christ, which is *us*.

Once we understand our primary gifts found in Romans, we then can understand the direction our life takes with the other gifts found in 1 Corinthians and Ephesians. When you truly seek God, you will listen to Him as He reveals the direction in which He wants you to go. Of course, free will comes into play. I *choose* to play the game. God is my coach. I can either obey what He asks of me or be disobedient and sit on the bench. The choice is mine. So how do the gifts in Romans lead us in the direction of our gifts in 1 Corinthians and Ephesians?

1 Corinthians 12:1–11 states: **"Now about spiritual gifts, brothers, I do not want you to be ignorant. You know that when you were pagans, somehow or other you were influenced and led astray to mute idols. Therefore I tell you that no one who is speaking by the Spirit of God says, 'Jesus be cursed,' and no one can say, 'Jesus is Lord,' except by the Holy Spirit. There are different kinds of gifts, but the same Spirit. There are different kinds of service, but the same Lord. There are different kinds of working, but the same God works all of them in all men. Now to each one the manifestation of the Spirit is given for the common good. To one there is given through the Spirit the message of wisdom, to another the message of knowledge by means of the same Spirit, to another faith by the same Spirit, to another gifts of healing by that one Spirit, to another miraculous powers, to another prophecy, to another distinguishing between spirits, to another speaking in different kinds of tongues, and to still another the interpretation of tongues. All these are the work of one and the same Spirit, and he gives them to each one, just as he determines."**

The gifts in Romans drive this next set of gifts because God has a purpose for each of us, a direction He wants us to go, and a certain degree of service based on the gifts He has given us. Everyone who lays down his life for Christ has these gifts because everyone is in the body of Christ. Since not everyone believes in Christ or lives according to His will, these gifts remain unrealized, dormant, and stifled. As we grow in the Lord and believe in Him with all of our mind, heart, soul, and strength, and understand the value God puts on us, we learn to accept our gifts graciously and learn how to use them for His glory. But before we do anything, we first must know who we are as a son or daughter of God.

The message in 1 Corinthians tells us that each of us has different gifts, different works, and different service. Just because we have the gift of wisdom or knowledge doesn't mean that we have to go into ministry. Nor does having the gift of prophecy or being able to discern good from evil mean that we have to go into ministry. What it does mean is that each of us is called to use our gifts according to our faith in every situation we face. Our whole life, how we live and love every day, is our greatest ministry. Remember that the Holy Spirit will show you what your gifts are. Though you have all of them, one or two will be shown to you as a primary gift. Once the Spirit reveals your gift, then God will show you how the gifts in Romans lead into the gifts listed in 1 Corinthians. A road map of your life starts to appear. Your life begins to make sense. The dots on your map start to line up to tell you why and where you have been, why and where you are, and why and where you are going. God wants to give you direction. He knows the perfect plans He has for you. He wants to lead you to a place where you can serve people according to your gifts.

The next set of gifts are the fivefold gifts of ministry. For those who feel God pulling and tugging and nudging them into further, more responsible acts of service, God has given further gifts, the gifts found in Ephesians 4:7–13. God isn't merely going to say you belong in ministry. He has set it up so that the gifts found in Romans and 1 Corinthians motivate and lead into a higher calling so your life's direction can be established.

In Ephesians 4:7–13 the Apostle Paul writes: "**But to each one of us grace has been given as Christ apportioned it. This is why it says: 'When he ascended on high, he led captives in his train and gave gifts to men (and women).' (What does 'he ascended' mean except that he also descended to the lower, earthly regions? He who descended is the very one who ascended higher than all the heavens, in order to fill the whole universe.) It was he who gave some (gifts) to be apostles, some to be prophets, some to be evangelists, and some to be pastors and teachers, to prepare God's people for works of service, so that the body of Christ may be built up until we all reach unity in the faith and in the knowledge of the Son of God and become mature, attaining to the whole measure of the fullness of Christ.**"

Though Christ came and saved us through His death and resurrection, we are still called to build up His church, which again is us. And He apportions gifts to ensure that this happens. It is up to us to use or misuse those gifts. Many people have a difficult time believing that God singles out individuals as apostles, prophets, evangelists, pastors, and teachers. Do we not limit ourselves in believing that we are *not* called to service through the gifts apportioned to us? Are we not *all* of these things and more when we truly submit ourselves to the obedience of Jesus Christ? The question is, Who are you? If you truly feel called to a greater act of service, know that you have been given these same gifts, and that through prayer, faith, and obedience, the Holy Spirit will reveal Himself to you. Why do you think the way you do? Where do you get your amazing drive and determination to help people? How is it that you are so quick to learn and so quick to comprehend? How is it that you have felt God's hand pushing you in directions you don't understand? Why at times have you felt so miserable living in the world and being of the world? Why have you been establishing your value as a man or woman from the world and what you *do* in it rather than believing what God says in James 1:17, "**Every good and perfect gift is from above, coming down from the Father of the heavenly lights, who does not change like shifting shadows.**"

Let God tell you who you are in the body of Jesus Christ because it is there that your value is determined and the mission for your life is established…should you choose to accept it. Before you *do* anything for God, you must first *be* the amazing man or woman you already are. It doesn't begin with "doing" anything; it begins by "being" you. Being you establishes your value and obedience will follow.

Once we learn of our gifts, should we publicly profess who we are? Absolutely not. I have shared my gifts and who I am in the body of Christ with very few people on this earth. Why? Because Satan will do everything he can to hit us with pride, arrogance, conceit, and judgment. And that is why we are told in Romans 12:3, **"For by the grace given me I say to every one of you: Do not think of yourself more highly than you ought, but rather think of yourself with sober judgment, in accordance with the measure of faith God has given you."** We did not appoint these gifts to ourselves. They were appointed to us by He who is in us through the Holy Spirit who gives so generously. It is with somber humility that I accept who I am, who Christ tells me I am. **"For everyone who exalts himself will be humbled, and he who humbles himself will be exalted"** (Luke 14:11). This is true of every one of us. As we humble ourselves in the Lord, He will pour out His Spirit into us and use the amazing gifts He has given us. He will use our talents and abilities as a platform for our gifts of the Spirit to help and serve people. In the world, Jesus was a carpenter. That is what He did for a living, but who He was in the Spirit was the Son of God. The Apostles were fishermen, tax collectors, and tent makers.

He is eager yet patient as you are finding out who you really are—who God Himself says you are. Not everyone is an apostle (builder of the church). Not everyone is a prophet (someone to whom God makes known a message for his people that is appropriate to their particular need or purpose). Not everyone is an evangelist (one who reaches out and naturally inspires and helps others in their testimony). Not everyone is or will be a pastor (one who shepherds the church by teaching the gospel).   Though some people are born teachers and seek that profession accordingly, I think we all have in us a gift of teaching. If you are a mother or father, you know this to be true on some level. See, that wasn't so bad. So many of us consider these gifts scary or irrelevant in the modern church. When we break down the gifts and understand them in our language, it is much easier to see that they are a part of each one of us who follows Christ. The body of Christ is *you* and *me*, all of us working together. Are you an active member and know who you are? Let Christ show you. He loves you so much!

"Dear Heavenly Father, let us not love with words or tongue but with actions and in truth" (1 John 3:18). Help us put our faith into action and give us the *Courage to Change*. Thank You for the wisdom and knowledge you have given us to move forward according to Your will. Help us remove ourselves from our own will and to listen to that inner voice of Your Holy Spirit that will lead us, break us, mold us, and transform us. Show us who we are and the amazing gifts You have given all of us. Give us the strength of an army of mighty warriors and the gentleness of a rose petal. Nurture us, discipline us, prune us, and show us the way. In the name of Jesus Christ I pray, Amen.

For Reflection:

What gift/s do you have to offer to the Body of Christ?

_____

_____

Beginning right now, how will you use that gift/s to contribute to the health of the Body of Christ?

_____

_____

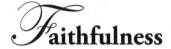aithfulness

"A call to action"

In the early spring of 2003 I gave my first "Faith in Action" seminar to the leadership staff of a large church in Pantego, Texas. They invited me to give a team-building seminar for all the staff of the church. It was my first official Faith in Action seminar. After I introduced Faith in Action, I began the seminar by placing numerous paper towels on the wooden stage, the very pulpit the pastor preached from every Sunday. The leadership of the church, along with the head pastor, sat in the congregation seats. As I finished placing the towels all over the floor, I pulled out a carton of eggs. I took one out and held it firmly in my hand. "There must be a lot of prayer warriors in here," I told the leaders, "and the prayer and faith in this room must be over the top, since you are the ones running the church, the shepherds of the church members." Then I asked them to focus on the egg and pray their hardest that as I dropped it from my waist, the egg wouldn't break.

So they began to pray, but what do you think happened? The egg splattered all over the paper towels, all over the stage. But how could that happen? How could the egg break if the leadership of the church was praying for it not to break? I pulled out another egg and repeated the same question, "What is it going to take to keep this egg from breaking when I drop it to the floor?" So I dropped the second one. Again the egg smashed against the floor, leaving more of a mess than the first one. This went on and on. "Come on now, aren't you guys praying? Where is your faith?" I asked. Finally, I had the last egg in my hand and I asked once more, "What is it going to take for this egg not to explode when I drop it to the floor?" And just as I was going to drop the last egg, a man got out of his seat, walked up to the stage, and physically took the egg from my hand. *Bravo!* He put his faith into action and proved the point of the exercise. The man stepped forward and proved that his faith was a call to action!

I looked deep into the eyes of each person sitting there and asked them how many times they had been the eggs that were dropped? How many times in their life had they felt broken like the eggs on the floor? I also asked them how many times they had been the ones who had dropped and cracked the eggs because they failed to take action? The huge auditorium was silent. The eyes of each person were big and round as I showed them that each one of them was precious and just as fragile as the egg, and without action accompanying their faith, they would sometimes break. Jesus makes all things new and restores our brokenness, but it is in our physical walk with Him that He can do His work in us.

The afternoon was just getting started. The next exercise was the "trust fall," where each church leader actually took a turn as the egg falling to the earth. Each person became responsible for the life and physical health of the others when he fell. Most of the leaders experienced nervousness, anxiety, and fear. I could hear the self-doubt, negativity, and fear sweep through the auditorium. The once quiet room was now filled with second-guessing, murmurs of fear, and some cries of hopelessness. Many of the leaders were obese, and almost all were out of shape and not physically confident. But how could this be? This was the leadership of a major church to which people came for direction in their lives. How could the very ones responsible for people's lives not be confident in and responsible for their own lives? The answer was easy. Each church leader was still just a person like everyone else and had to conquer fear just like everyone else—the hard way. Even church leaders, sometimes more than others, put so much focus on others that they forget about their own lives, their own physical needs and passions. Sure, serving others entails self-sacrifice, but some sacrifice isn't sacrifice at all—it is sometimes ignorance or avoidance of taking care of ourselves.

I then had them form two lines below the rather high stage and taught everyone how to lock their arms and position their bodies. They had to learn because they would soon have a life in their hands as they caught each falling person (the fragile egg). The drop was substantial. The feet of the person falling backward off the stage were eye level with the tallest man, who was about 6' 3".

One by one I would bring each person to the edge and ask him about something he had been struggling with. To my surprise, the leaders of this church had many of the same issues that all of us face: finances, children, divorce, and even abusive relationships. One rugged man's eyes filled with tears as I reminded him that his finances had nothing to do with his value as a man. I shared with him that God would give him wisdom and direction regarding his finances, but that God placed absolutely no value on his ability or inability to provide financially for his family. Just then I asked him to attach the fear in his finances to the fall and allow God to strengthen him during the physical act of falling and trusting that he would be caught. With tears rolling down his face, he literally put his fear of finances on the altar and physically plunged blindly backward into the vast unknown. The fear of falling became his fear of finances as he fell, and the physical action he took in response to the faith he had in his Father in heaven broke the yoke of that fear. His peers caught him; he was safe. He didn't break like the egg but emerged stronger in his faith and trust in God.

The day was about to get even more interesting. About halfway through the trust fall, a young girl came running into the large sanctuary and shouted, "Come quick, the youth center is on fire!" Everyone sat frozen for a second and looked at each other and at me, thinking it might be part of my team-building exercise. Well, it wasn't. I was a little off-the-wall at times, but I certainly wasn't into burning down buildings as an object lesson! So we dropped what we were doing and ran across the church campus to see what the commotion was all about. Sure enough, black smoke was coming out of the youth building. By the time I got there, one of the men had already been inside and found a trash can that was in flames. He knew exactly where a fire extinguisher was and put the blaze out himself. The main room of the youth center was completely engulfed in smoke. The fire crew got there and the building was saved from any major damage. As we were out talking about what had happened, many of the church staff came nonchalantly walking up the sidewalk just talking, laughing, and joking around. They had just assumed that someone else would take care of the problem and hadn't actively gotten involved. Interestingly enough, they were the very ones not taking the seminar seriously either. Amazing how that works….

We made our way back into the auditorium. I felt the Holy Spirit so strongly because the fire in the youth center had just proved what faith in action was all about. We can't just walk around being spiritual all the time and say we love ourselves and others. We absolutely at all times must accompany our faith with action, otherwise, youth centers get burned down and sometimes youth with them. As I showed them the significance of the fiery youth center, I asked them all a few questions, "How much more valuable are *you* than that building? Where else in your life do you let others handle problems and not get involved? Where else in your life do you not put your faith into action?" Once again it was so quiet in the large room that you could hear each person breathing.

So who put out the fire? I wouldn't be surprised if God himself lit that fire to prove His point. The man who was the first to get to the youth center and put out the fire was the same man who had earlier gotten out of his seat and taken the egg from my hand. He was the very man who had contacted me and scheduled the seminar in the first place. He was a man of action not because it was the right thing to do but because his faith in God was accompanied by action.

The ordeal with the youth center ate up a lot of time, and many of the church leaders had to get back to their duties. We ended the seminar with five people left, the very ones who hadn't taken it seriously. They finally tapped in and wanted to overcome their fear. Not coincidentally, they were also the ones who were obese. But they stayed and mustered up the courage to fall, the *Courage to Change*. They found the courage to begin the process of putting their faith into action. Everyone in the seminar learned the importance of being physically healthy and its role in putting their faith into action. **Physical exercise is a daily and weekly active "trust fall" that puts action to your faith and helps you overcome spiritual obstacles, the very obstacles that keep you from being healthy.**

Before you can be faithful in anything, however, *you must first be faithful to God*. Before you can be faithful to God, you must understand *His* faithfulness to *you*. The *Life Application Journal* is designed to expose you to the faithfulness of God. As you journal and learn to ask Him for things, you will see how His faithfulness is perfect by how He answers you *with His actions*.

In James 2:17 we are told, **"Faith by itself, if it is not accompanied by action, is dead."** Why is this significant? It shows us the very nature of God's faithfulness to us. His faithfulness is perfect. He always does what He says He is going to do. His faithfulness to you is always followed with action. When you realize how faithful God is you will become faithful to Him in all you do—including taking care of yourself.

Every story, every lesson, every prayer, and every truth in the Bible is backed with God's faithfulness to us by His actions. Every thought and every command Jesus ever taught was accompanied with action. He didn't just *talk about* healing the sick, He healed the sick. He didn't just *talk about* raising Lazarus from the dead, He raised him from the dead. He didn't just *talk about* love, He lived it every moment He was with us. He didn't just *talk about* dying on a cross and coming back to us on the third day, He actually died on a cross and rose again on the third day. His faithfulness to us is perfect, lacking nothing.

As we speak things into existence with faith, hope, love, and the authority of Jesus Christ, our actions must follow every time. In Proverbs 20:11 we see that **"even a child is known by his actions, by whether his conduct is pure and right."** We aren't known by what we say, but by what we do for ourselves and others with action.

"You see that a person is justified by what he does and not by faith alone."
(James 2:24)

Why is a person justified by what he does and not by faith alone? Because it is in the very nature of God to take action, and since we are created in His image, we too have in our essence the need to act.

Action is at our very core, a part of us whether we accept it or not. When we do not truly love ourselves and others with action, we deprive ourselves and others of one of our most basic functions as God's children. It is impossible to separate faith from action. It is impossible to separate love from action. It is impossible to separate prayer from action, dreams from action, or goals from action. Thus it is impossible to separate our physical health from action. **"They claim to know God, but by their actions they deny Him. They are detestable, disobedient, and unfit for doing anything good"** (Titus 1:16). Our actions show how much we love God. Our actions prove what is in our hearts as well as what is *not*.

We also find in James 2:22 that **"Our Faith is made complete by what we do."** It is made complete by living the way we were designed, by taking action. How many of you have fervently prayed for God to heal your bodies, yet done nothing to change your lifestyle and continue eating candy and high fattening foods? How many prayers are said from the couch instead of the treadmill or stationary bike? How many of you have prayed earnestly for God to heal someone else's body, yet done nothing to encourage them to change their lifestyle by taking action? The proper thing to do for someone like this is take them a casserole of some kind, candied yams with marshmallows, or several pies, right! Wrong! **How can we expect God to answer the requests and prayers that are formed out of our own disregard for life?** How can we exercise our faith and expect Him to heal our body of lifestyle-induced diseases if we do absolutely nothing to change our lifestyles by taking action? If we are living with God in our hearts, our actions accompany His actions because we are working together as Father and son or daughter. I for one want to please my Father in heaven by taking care of His most basic gift to me—my physical body.

James 2:15–16 tells us: **"Suppose a brother or sister is without clothes and daily food. If one of you says to him, 'Go, I wish you well; keep warm and well fed' but does nothing about his physical needs, what good is it?"** It is your actions here that are needed to help a brother or sister. But what exactly are you doing when you give this person food and clothing? Are you not helping her preserve the life given her? Are you not giving food so that she won't starve to death? Are you not giving her clothing to keep her from freezing to death? The same action meant for our brothers and sisters is also meant for ourselves. Are we not just as valuable as our brothers and sisters? Are we not called to love them as ourselves? We give others food, clothing, and shelter with love, yet we go back inside and kill ourselves with cigarettes, drugs, alcohol, and complacency.

I encourage you, my brother and my sister, to put your faith into action. Go to the source of all motivation and act as Christ would act. Put your faith to work as you know that God is putting His faithfulness to work for you!

For Reflection:

Are there some areas of your life in which you have not been putting your faith into action?

_____

_____

What can you do right now—and for the rest of this week—to put your faith into action?

_____

_____

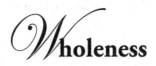holeness

"The feeling of completeness found in following and loving Jesus Christ"

I used to think it was up to me to balance my life and the things in it. I would do my best to balance my job, friends, family, God, recreation, working out, and a whole slew of things. The original name of this program was "Balanced Energies." I realized over time that I had it all wrong about how I was to balance my life and the things in it. I learned that God is not something that I balance in my life. I learned that everything in my life that I had to balance—such as my job, writing books, friends, family, recreation, working out, relaxation, and even ministry—was in the world, but it was God who was the fulcrum on which everything balanced. I no longer balance God with the things I do in my life. How could I possibly put God in the same category and figure out how to fit Him into my busy schedule as I do everything else?

Instead, all the things I do in my life are balanced *on* God. He provides the way and tells me if I am off-balance with too much work and not enough play. He tells me if I am putting too much emphasis on working out and if I am being vain with my fitness. He tells me if I am relying on my wife and family too much to help me with my stress instead of using Him as my refuge. So why am I using the word *balance* in a section on wholeness?

At one time or another we have all thought about or desired more balance in our lives, something to help us put everything in perspective. Balance is definitely something we are all called to find—but is there something that must come first to help us find that balance? I believe ultimately that we are all seeking wholeness more than balance. It is wholeness that tells us what to balance, what is important, and what drives us. But what is wholeness? **Wholeness comes from the same root word as *Holiness*, and it means "complete, lacking nothing."** Our heavenly Father is holy, lacking nothing. He is pure, complete in every way. His holiness is wholeness, and He will show us how to be filled with His truth and His purpose. The events and things we do in life are what we balance, but these are largely dictated by our wholeness. If you don't have joy in your heart, how can you balance work time with family time? If you don't have the peace of our Lord in your heart and take it with you wherever you go, how do you expect to add an exercise program into your life without getting overwhelmed? It simply becomes "one more thing in your life" that you are "balancing" instead of seeking wholeness or holiness by a moment-by-moment loving, intimate relationship with Jesus Christ.

Without Jesus Christ, you will never experience the true joy in everything you do because *true joy comes from Him*. We can experience good things on our own, but they will simply be experiences, nothing more, a perception of reality. But with a living, loving God reigning in our hearts, we become more than we are. We become whole or holy, lacking nothing. And since we all fall short of the glory of God, it is Christ's forgiveness that perfects and completes our wholeness, thus enabling us to balance whatever comes our way in life. God will equip us with the wisdom to problem-solve and balance each day. He will teach us how to love ourselves and how to love others as ourselves.

We have gotten away from loving ourselves. We have spent so much time serving others, doing for others, loving others, and focusing outward that we have lost our sense of what God intended in saying, **"Love your neighbor as yourself,"** the second great commandment. How can we truly love others if we are not whole, do not understand our true value and purpose in life, and fall prey to complacency, insecurities, and depression? We often think that antidepressant drugs will cure the problem or that a two-week vacation will do the trick. They may help, but ultimately they have nothing to do with our wholeness. They will not—cannot—give us peace, joy, and true deliverance from the stresses this world puts on us.

The Holy Bible is very clear about the holiness of God. But what *is* Holiness and how do we attain it? Through my studies, I have discovered that in every context in the Bible where the holiness of God and men is mentioned, one thing is present—one thing that always and without fail accompanies holiness: ACTION. Referring to when the Israelites watched in amazement as God protected them from certain death from Pharaoh by closing the sea over their Egyptian pursuers, Exodus 15:10–13 tells us:

> **"But you blew with your breath, and the sea covered them. They sank like lead in the mighty waters. Who among the gods is like you, O LORD? Who is like you—majestic in holiness, awesome in glory, working wonders? You stretched out your right hand and the earth swallowed them. In your unfailing love, you will lead the people you have redeemed. In your strength, you will guide them to your holy dwelling."**

God is holy because He not only talks a good talk but He follows every promise with action. He "works wonders." "But you blew with your breath, and the sea covered them" states the physical action God took to protect His people. God's promises always come with an action because He is a faithful God. He does what He says He is going to do, which is led by an unfailing love and integrity that is perfect, whole, and lacking nothing. So His actions are also whole and perfect. "You stretched out your right hand and the earth swallowed them." God doesn't just *tell us* He loves us. He shows us through His faithfulness as we let Him lead our lives. "In your unfailing love, you will lead the people you have redeemed. In your strength, you will guide them to your holy dwelling." God doesn't have strength; He *is* strength. He doesn't just have power, He *is* almighty and all-powerful and shows us with action.

And here is the clincher. God was there to protect them from the sea and the Pharaoh as they walked through, yes. But they had to *walk through*. There was no way around it. Can you imagine how they must have felt looking up at a roaring wall of water thousands of feet high on both sides, totally vulnerable and at the mercy of God, while looking behind them and seeing a wall of fire falling from the sky between them and the Pharaoh? But they walked through anyway. Their action absolutely had to accompany God's action. God will not do it for us. He can, but He won't, because He wants you and me to love ourselves and others with action by our own free will.

God's way is holy because He will never tire in His pursuit of our hearts. He will always take action to see that we are safe and in His will. Even God's discipline comes from His holiness because He is simply fulfilling a promise to us never to leave us nor forsake us, to always have our best intentions in His mind and on His heart, always and without fail loving us. The prophet Isaiah makes reference to a highway we must walk on to keep us holy:

> **"And a highway will be there; it will be called the Way of Holiness. The unclean will not journey on it; it will be for those who walk in that Way; wicked fools will not go about on it. No lion will be there, nor will any ferocious beast get up on it; they will not be found there. But only the redeemed will walk there, and the ransomed of the LORD will return. They will enter Zion with singing; everlasting joy will crown their heads. Gladness and joy will overtake them, and sorrow and sighing will flee away."** (Isaiah 35:8–10)

There is a physical journey we must travel as we live in the grace of God, and the more closely we stay on the right path, or this highway that Isaiah shows us, the more holy we become. "But only the redeemed will walk there, and the ransomed of the LORD will return." Isaiah is prophetically speaking of Jesus here because Jesus has redeemed us from our sins, and as we follow Him, we walk in love in all things and our wholeness is made complete. But we all must realize that at all times the action associated with holiness is *physical*. 2 Corinthians 7:1 states: **"Since we have these promises, dear friends, let us purify ourselves from everything that contaminates body and spirit, perfecting holiness out of reverence for God."** Come on, Church body, how do we purify ourselves from everything that contaminates body and spirit without action? Do we just pray for God to deliver us, or do we take action? Physical exercise and good nutrition purify us by burning out impurities stored up in our bodies. It makes us strong and resilient. The action we take in exercise also battles complacency and fear and helps us live as warriors instead of slaves: **"But now that you have been set free from sin and have become slaves to God, the benefit you reap leads to holiness, and the result is eternal life"** (Romans 6:22). The reason "the benefit you reap leads to holiness" is that your faith and acceptance of Jesus Christ into your heart must be accompanied by action. Being a slave to God means being a slave to love, peace, joy, and hope. How awesome is that? How many of you want just one of those? **As you grow closer to the Lord with your actions that lead to holiness, He will use you in proportion to your walk with Him.** Walking with the Lord doesn't mean walking around in a daze all day just loving the Lord. **Walking with the Lord means building relationships with people based on how much love you have for yourself through your understanding of how much God loves you.** And this is how you love others as yourself.

We are told in 1 John 3:18, **"Dear children, let us not love with words or tongue but with actions and in truth."** Do you think John is telling us to exclude ourselves from these wise words from God? Are we supposed to love only *other people* with action and truth? No, if we are to love our neighbor as ourselves, it is high time we first start loving ourselves with action and in truth. And this means knowing ourselves, knowing what God says about us individually. If we would just listen, He will tell each of us how much He loves us and what His plans are for us. I will prophetically speak this truth to every person who reads this, and every person who doesn't, all across this great planet. One of the greatest desires God has is for you to be healthy individually and corporately as the body of Christ. Our heavenly Father weeps every day as He sees the sickness and disease caused by our lack of physical action. He sees us day after day put junk into our bodies and then do nothing to burn it off or **"purify ourselves from everything that contaminates body and spirit"** (2 Corinthians 7:1). Treating our bodies with respect with action and in truth is a crucial and widely overlooked part of reaching wholeness or holiness in our life. Physical exercise and taking care of ourselves is simply a catalyst for putting our faith in action, loving ourselves and others with action.

As we are told "it is better to give than to receive," we must look deeply into what this really means. Loving ourselves with action is not receiving anything at all. Receiving is what we accept from someone else. In this context it is absolutely better to give than to receive. But loving ourselves with action is a *gift to ourselves, from ourselves,* to honor God. Let me repeat that. **Loving ourselves with action is a gift to ourselves, from ourselves, to honor God.** As we take the time to exercise and eat right, we **give** to ourselves and honor God with our bodies. We also give to others by showing them that we love ourselves enough to take action. We are telling others that we do matter and are important and can show the fruit that action produces by way of decreased sickness and disease, increased energy and enthusiasm, strength, stamina, and endurance, all of which are needed as we love and serve others with action.

Once you feel the love of God pouring through you and act accordingly by clothing yourself with Jesus Christ, then you will reach a sense of wholeness or holiness. Hebrews 12:10–14 states, **"Make every effort to live in peace with all men and to be holy; without holiness, no one will see the Lord."** The bottom line is that *in your obedience you will find wholeness* because God fills you with His truth as you walk in love. He will drive out what is unclean and unwanted and will replace it with Himself, the source of all that is holy. It may hurt a little as He does this, but the rewards are victory and freedom.

For Reflection:

What are three actions you can take right now to love yourself and secure wholeness in your life?

_____

_____

It is better to give than to receive. So, when you love yourself (act kindly toward yourself), are you giving or receiving?

_____

_____

IMAGE OF GOD

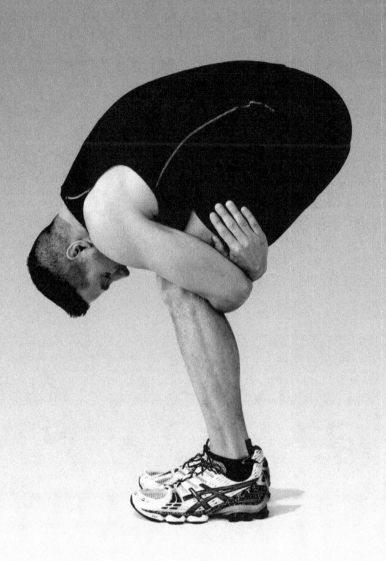

"Then God said, Let us make man in our image, in our likeness, and let them rule over the fish of the sea and the birds of the air, over the livestock, over all the earth, and over all the creatures that move along the ground." So God created him; male and female he created them.

WEEK TWELVE

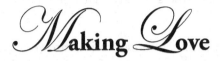

Making Love

"The single greatest expression of God's love shared between a husband and wife"

Why in the world would I have a section on making love in a book on health? That's easy! Because it is the *only* time in the human experience when a person's body, mind, emotions, attitude, actions, and spirit are in harmony with each other and become one with another person. Your physical health and the spiritual behavior behind it is what will make lovemaking either a beautiful, sacred experience, or an insecure, scary one. Throughout my career I have seen how closely related this topic is to a person's health.

In Genesis 1:28, God's first commandment to us is **"to be fruitful and multiply."** It is primal and at the very core of why we were created. **Making love is the single greatest act of God's love between husband and wife and must be experienced in its proper design for you to truly understand the beauty and respect of the body God gave you.** Making love is the most vulnerable you will ever be and is the most intimate act of love you will ever physically and emotionally experience. It is the greatest and only time where every part of your being is experienced at the same time—your body, mind, emotions, spirit, and everything in between. At no other time is there such harmony within yourself and your body and with another person. You must trust and be trusted by your spouse on a level not experienced anywhere else in your relationship. Respect, honor, and gentleness should be present on a level far exceeding any other point in your life. It is the closest that two people will ever get to experiencing the fullness of God's love with another person.

> **"Therefore, I urge you, brothers, in view of God's mercy, to offer your bodies as living sacrifices, holy and pleasing to God—this is your spiritual act of worship."** (Romans 12:1)

God knows that it is impossible to separate your body from your spirit. He created them to work together. They are coexisting or working in harmony together, or against each other, at all times. This scripture tells you a little about how you are to offer yourself to your spouse, not just to God. Part of how you offer your body as a living sacrifice, holy and pleasing to God, is how you offer yourself to your spouse. If you offer forgiveness and the grace of Christ to each other, why would it be any different to offer your bodies to each other as holy and pleasing to God? It is your spiritual act of worship.

To illustrate my point, think of Christmas when you see beautiful presents under the tree. Each present is carefully wrapped and dolled up with ribbon, lace, and a decorative label. The present

275

itself is beautiful. It is carefully and strategically placed under the tree with other presents to make one beautiful Christmas scene. It is difficult to even open all the presents because of how intricately they are wrapped, the time and care that went into them, and the tree that looks so bare without them.

Here is my question to you. How much more precious are you as a beautiful gift to your spouse than that present under the tree? Isn't your gift of "you" worth far more care and attention than the appearance of a package under the tree? What you outwardly unwrap and experience together as you make love is the result of the hidden treasure found inside the present, the actual gift the package protects, your love for one another.

You see, though the presents look beautiful under the tree, it is what is inside that is of far more value than the package itself. But the whole experience of Christmas involves unwrapping something outwardly beautiful to find the "pearl" on the inside, a gift from the heart inspired by the love and joy of Jesus Christ. **And that is why taking care of yourself, and physically and sexually offering yourself to each other, is the outward expression of your inner beauty and godliness.**

Present yourselves to each other as confident, sensual, and sexy individuals with lean, strong, and healthy bodies; not *perfect* bodies, but realistic healthy bodies. 1 Corinthians 7:3 says, **"The husband should fulfill his marital duty to his wife, and likewise the wife to her husband."** God wants you to please each other—and *often!*

"The wife's body does not belong to her alone but also to her husband. In the same way, the husband's body does not belong to him alone but also to his wife" (1 Corinthians 7:4). This is all the more reason to offer yourself as a radiant gift to each other.

"Do not deprive each other except by mutual consent and for a time, so that you may devote yourselves to prayer. Then come together again so that Satan will not tempt you because of your lack of self-control" (1 Corinthians 7:5). God shows here that what He designs is pleasure between husband or wife is not merely procreation. So, if your lovemaking isn't a physically exhausting event, then I might suggest . . . *well anyway!* The act itself of making love is very physical and requires both of you to be healthy and to learn how your bodies move together. What feels good? Learn together. A strong, healthy body actually brings out the gentleness and physical sensitivity needed to best please each other. You can focus more on the love between you rather than the fact that your lungs are going to explode from overexertion.

In essence you should want to offer yourself to your husband or wife as a lean, healthy, and toned gift, not as a "perfect specimen," or anything unrealistic, but as a healthy and vibrant gift. Your body is the elegant gift box, which holds the pearl inside. Enjoy your bodies with each other for the rest of your long, healthy lives!

So why wait until marriage to make love?

Is this an outdated principle or is it an age-old principle that God designed to preserve the holiness of where He is taking you, the precious beauty of becoming one with someone in a loving covenant relationship? Only one person is worthy of unwrapping your present and finding the pearl—your gentle, loving, and committed husband or wife. It is truly beautiful.

I struggled with this principle for a long time. But I felt God's love calling me to a greater level of commitment, a greater level of obedience through my love affair with Him. When I surrendered this part of my life, I was shown a woman's true beauty—physically, mentally, emotionally, and spiritually. As I honored God with my body in this way, then *and only then* did I open myself to my wife, the woman God handpicked for me, Silesia. And it was her heart that further convicted me to be the honorable man I was designed to be. I remember the exact event that set this commitment in stone.

At the beginning of our courtship, though we had never been sexually intimate, a few times Silesia and I allowed ourselves to get too aroused without being married. I remember Silesia asking me if I was worried if we would have sex or not. And with a confident boast, I told her that, no, I wasn't worried about it and that we weren't going to have sex before marriage. But then she said, "How can you say that when it has been so intense and amazing this far?" It hit me like a freight train running over my head as the Holy Spirit convicted me even further. If she had any doubt whatsoever of my intentions, or had any doubt or worry about having sex, then I wasn't honoring her the way God designed me to. It is *my* job to protect her heart, and since her body is intricately connected to her spirit, I must honor and protect her body as well. After all, I had no rights to her body until we were married. A woman's body is absolutely connected to her heart, her emotions, and her spirit, and anything that violates her body will undoubtedly affect all the other parts of her. It is my duty as a man to protect not only her heart, emotions, and spirit, but her body as well because they are all connected. Though it was up to me to take the lead in setting boundaries regarding physical and sexual intimacy, Silesia did as well. In this way we honored each other.

For a while, as I still lived in Dallas, Silesia and the kids would come up from Houston to visit me for the weekend. But did we stay together? Absolutely not. I slept in my gym with a sleeping bag and exercise mat or in my car. Before we were married, I was closing on a house in north Houston. I still had an apartment in Dallas but was staying with Silesia at her apartment 40 miles north of where we now live. This lasted for three months as I finalized everything with the house. But wait, though I trained clients and spent the day with Silesia and kids during the day, every night for three months I slept in my car out in the parking lot. It was the dead of winter and got down to 19 degrees, but it was by far more important to me to honor Silesia. Many people say it would have been fine for me to sleep on the couch. But the Bible says to stay away from *even the appearance of evil.* Shelby and Matthew needed to see their mother honored and respected, something they had never seen before. But in reality, have you seen my wife? Yeah, right! Sleeping on the couch would have led to disaster. Though my whole being craved her, God's love was more powerful, and the honor He poured into my heart overpowered any physical desire I had for her. Believe me—it wasn't easy. Having the grounds keeper chain me to the steering wheel of my vehicle each night also helped! Just kidding...maybe!

We were engaged on Thanksgiving Day 2004. After finally closing on the house, I moved in January 2005. We still had until March 25 to get married, so I lived in the house alone. But I still wanted our wedding bed to be undefiled and unslept in until our wedding night. So even though we picked out our bedroom set and mattress and put the bedroom together, I slept downstairs in a guest bedroom until our wedding night. Only then did God give me access to Silesia and Silesia to me. God gave us an amazing love story that began with honor, respect, and surrender to Him.

Just as I once did, how many of you still freely give your bodies over to sexual desire or somehow use sex in a way other than the way it was designed in a marital relationship? I have seen and also experienced firsthand the hurt from the brokenness of premarital sexual relationships and cohabitation. It damages not only your spirit but your body as well because they are connected.

1 Corinthians 6:18–20 states, **"Flee from sexual immorality. All other sins a man commits are outside his body, but he who sins sexually sins against his own body."** I used to think that this meant abusive sex, multiple partners, orgies, or extramarital affairs. I didn't realize that I was doing the same thing by having sex with a girlfriend, even if I *thought* I loved her. I dishonored myself and her and created a bond between the two of us that should exist only with my wife. I, in essence, had sex with another man's future wife. *Oh my!* By keeping a woman pure by honoring her in this way, I also honor her future husband if that person is not me!

After training a client one day in Irving, Texas, I wondered how I could teach the importance of honoring a woman in this way so that people—especially people of the male gender—would understand. I felt compelled to walk outside, so I did. To my left was beautiful landscaping with flowers, mulch, plants, and decorative benches. I was drawn to the freshly planted flowers and went over to them. Virtually every color was visible to my eye, and the smell was incredible. I felt God nudging me to touch and smell one more closely in order to fully experience its beauty. But as I bent down to pick one of the flowers, I realized that there were two ways for me to experience it. The first way involved reaching down and picking one. I could bring it to my level to observe its beautiful smell and silken petals. But when I thought of this, I realized that to do so would take its life in the process. The first way was selfish and disrespectful to the flower, not to mention the person or company that paid for the flower to be put there. To get what I wanted, I had to kill the flower. The thought made me feel horrible. So I got down on my knees, on its level, and bent way down so my nose touched the petals. I took in a big breath and could smell its beautiful aroma. The petals were also soft and silky on my nose. Though my hands and knees got a little dirty, I realized that if I truly respected the beautiful flower I should preserve its life so that other people could also enjoy it as I had.

I realized just then: *How much more precious is a woman? How much more careful should I be to keep her rooted and safe?* See, the flower didn't actually belong to me, it belonged to God (and whoever owned the property). It was up to me, whether or not, to put its life before my own selfish wants. I realized that having sex outside of marriage was just like reaching down and uprooting the flower for my own gain, my own selfish desires. I realized that to get the woman of my dreams, I would need to honor her by putting her needs before my own, to treat her body as a precious rose worthy of respect and honor. I stood there in the parking lot for quite some time just staring at the flowers and thanking God for the beauty He showed me.

All this is to say that the more ways you learn to respect and honor your own body and the body of someone else, the greater appreciation and honor you will have for your health. Sexual purity comes with power, love, and respect for oneself, all of which you need as you regain your physical health. Please respect yourself and your future spouse by honoring God by remaining or becoming sexually pure. If your relationship did not start this way, you cannot go back, but it is never too late to change. And so you should. God is right there ready to forgive you and restore you and give you and your boyfriend, girlfriend or spouse a fresh start. All you have to do is ASK.

For Reflection:

As you take stock of the condition of your sexual wholeness, are there changes that need to be made in light of the truth shared in this section? Do you need to examine and, with God's help, change your attitudes about sexuality, your mate, and purity?

_____

_____

Do you need to pray right now for a fresh start in your sexuality?

_____

_____

Final Encouragement

Dear Friends:

I am so proud of you! It is almost time for graduation, a celebration of your hard work and breakthroughs. Now is when *Courage to Change* truly begins. It is time to put your faith in action! *You are* the program. *Be* the program. This book and *Life Application Journal* has taught you the importance of the "as yourself" part of the second great commandment, "Love your neighbor as yourself." Over the past 12 weeks, you have learned that how you take care of and love "you" directly affects your ability to love and serve others. Now it is time to spread the health! We need your help to spread the message and importance of this ministry.

As you have learned, a time of change is upon us. We are reminded in Matthew 28:19 of the Great Commission to **"not only make disciples of all nations by baptizing them in the name of the Father and of the Son and of the Holy Spirit, but to also teach them to obey everything Christ has commanded."** Being reborn through Christ and knowing the Bible is but the mere beginning of living a life for Christ.

Though the love and peace of Christ is very much alive, over the past 12 weeks, you have gotten a taste of how the body of Christ as a whole is riddled with complacency, obesity, sickness, fear, and insecurities. We need the message of the *Courage to Change* to spread. Help Silesia and I spread the raw beauty and power of helping others like you put their faith in action, beginning with the basics of good health practices.

Friends, we are in a time of great emptiness. The world is hungering for leadership. I feel great distress yet also a strong hope among our brothers and sisters. There has been—especially since 9/11—a deep hunger for truth among all nations. Those who are lost unknowingly search for Christ, and those who are saved search for more without knowing why. Their hearts yearn for something beyond themselves, but they do not know how to get it. The enemy knows that he can do nothing about our salvation once we give our lives to Christ, but what he *can* and *is* doing to the body of Christ is stealing our joy and keeping us from walking in the heritage and authority of God while we are here. Through our own actions of love and discipleship, we can appropriate and take back what is rightly ours, the abundant life that Jesus restored for us.

We are reminded in Acts 16:4 that **"as Paul and Silas traveled from town to town, they delivered the decisions reached by the Apostles and elders in Jerusalem for the people to obey. So the churches were strengthened in the Faith and grew daily in numbers."** The Lord will use this message to fill your seats on Sunday. Putting your faith in action creates loyalty to a church home and provides a spiritual covering for our families. I hear a cry for action from around the world. And this action-driven message of Christ begins in each and every Christ-follower on earth. To change the world, we must first change ourselves.

And as the believers, inspired by the Holy Spirit, reveal the truth of their actions of obedience, and their faith is made complete by what they do, your churches will be strengthened in the faith and grow daily in numbers. For in obedience there is loyalty through healthy living practices, tithing, creating lasting relationships and new ministries, and doing all the deeds that God has commanded. The greatest being that we "walk" in love. And that means *action!*

Let us look into our hearts, my brothers and sisters, and come together as leaders. The heart of *Courage to Change* begins with establishing or integrating *Courage to Change* Men's and Women's Leadership Teams within your churches, schools, companies, and sports facilities, and using the *Courage to Change* books and journals as a tool for putting your faith in action.

We know that without accountability to and from other Christ followers, we will never fulfill our own missions as children of the almighty God. **"Now we know that whatever the law says, it says to those who are under the law, so that every mouth may be silenced and the whole world be held accountable to God. Therefore, no one will be declared righteous in his sight by observing the law, rather, through the law we become conscious of sin"** (Romans 3:19–20). These member-facilitated leadership teams within your churches using the *Courage to Change* books and journals will provide the accountability necessary to create the healthy living that God desires in all of you. And the only way you become truly conscious of sin is by the support and accountability of other Christ-followers and by humbly asking God for His wisdom and direction. You then put your *faith in action* once you have the answer.

God will lovingly pull the truth out of you as you write in the *Courage to Change* journals. "As it is written, so shall it be done." The write-it-down process is the precursor to all other actions because your thoughts and prayers are brought to physical reality as you write them down. How can you do what you need to do if you keep everything in your head? Let it out. Write it down and free your mind of all things except positive thoughts as inspired by the word of God. Let your concerns out and give them away. Let God extract the truth from within you and write it down.

I feel a great urgency for all mankind to repent and spread as much love as possible in the form of action. Too often it seems we are doing the bare minimum for God. The time is near, the time is now to build the walls and ceiling of God's foundation by taking action. This foundation is the very ground on which we build our churches and homes and schools. Let's resolve not to let the storm fall in upon the foundation of God, for we are incomplete if we fail to take action to protect and keep alive the word of God inside all of us.

Have an amazing life full of purpose, smile as much as possible, and make healthy choices!

In Christ Jesus,

Brian Wellbrock
Faith in Action
www.courage2change.org
Helping you have the *Courage to Change!*